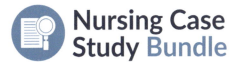

ACCESS 46 ADDITIONAL NURSING CASE STUDIES!

Unlock Your Critical Thinking through realistic scenarios in our nursing case studies...

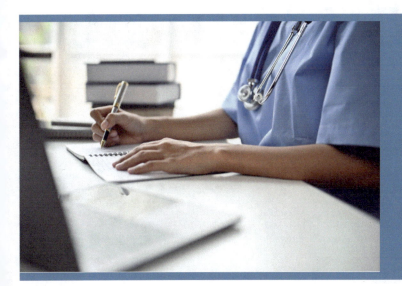

The Nursing Case Study Course Includes:

- 62 Case Study Lessons
- 271 Practice Questions
- 65 Cheat Sheets
- 44 Images
- 20 Mnemonics

Explore the Case Studies Course:
nursing.com/course/nursing-case-studies

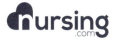

Nursing Case Study Bundle

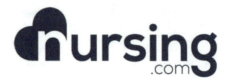

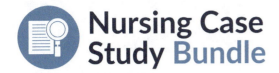

TABLE OF CONTENTS

CASE STUDIES:

Myocardial Infarction (MI)......1

Acute Kidney Injury (AKI)......11

Cirrhosis......17

COPD......23

Pneumonia......29

Stroke......35

Seizures......40

Diabetes Mellitus (DM)......45

Cushing's Disease......50

Burn Injury......55

Breast Cancer......60

Hyperthyroidism......68

Bipolar Disorder......75

Septic Shock......82

Maternal Newborn......89

Heart Failure......98

CHEAT SHEETS:

Right vs Left-Sided Heart Failure......104

Acute Kidney Injury Pathochart......105

Stroke Symptoms by Location......106

Steps to Critical Thinking......107

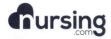

MYOCARDIAL INFARCTION (MI)

Nursing Case Study #1
(Myocardial Infarction)

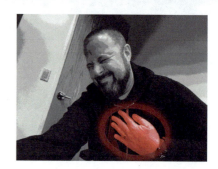

Pathophysiology:

A crucial aspect of comprehending myocardial infarction is exploring its pathophysiology. We will delve into the intricate details of how atherosclerosis, the buildup of plaque in coronary arteries, leads to the formation of blood clots and the subsequent interruption of blood flow to the heart muscle. This disruption in blood supply triggers a cascade of events, ultimately resulting in the death of cardiac cells.

Patient:

Mr. Salazar, a 57-year-old male, arrives at the Emergency Department (ED) with complaints of chest pain that began approximately one hour after dinner while he was working. He characterizes the discomfort as an intense "crushing pressure" located centrally in his chest, extending down his left arm and towards his back. He rates the pain's severity as 4/10. Upon examination, Mr. Salazar exhibits diaphoresis and pallor, accompanied by shortness of breath (SOB).

***Test your knowledge by referencing the answer key at the end of this study!*

Critical Thinking Check #1	*(Bloom's Taxonomy: Application)*
What further nursing assessments need to be performed for Mr. Salazar?	

Critical Thinking Check #2	*(Bloom's Taxonomy: Analysis)*
What interventions do you anticipate being ordered by the provider?	

NURSING.com - "Tools and Confidence to Succeed in Nursing School."
©2023 TazKai LLC | NURSING.com - Reproduction Strictly Prohibited
Disclaimer information at NURSING.com

MYOCARDIAL INFARCTION (MI)

Nursing Case Study #1
(Page 2)

Upon conducting a comprehensive assessment, it was observed that the patient exhibited no signs of jugular vein distention (JVD) or edema. Auscultation revealed normal heart sounds with both S1 and S2 present, while the lungs remained clear, albeit with scattered wheezes. The patient's vital signs were recorded as follows:

- **BP** 140/90 mmHg SpO2 90% on Room Air
- **HR** 92 bpm and regular Ht 173 cm
- **RR** 32 bpm Wt 104 kg
- **Temp** 36.9°C

The 12-lead EKG report indicated the presence of "Normal sinus rhythm (NSR) with frequent premature ventricular contractions (PVCs) and three- to four-beat runs of ventricular tachycardia (VT)." Additionally, there was ST-segment elevation in leads I, aVL, and V2 through V6 (3-4mm), accompanied by ST-segment depression in leads III and aVF.

Cardiac enzyme levels were collected but were awaiting results at the time of assessment. A chest x-ray was also ordered to provide further diagnostic insights.

In response to the patient's condition, the healthcare provider prescribed the following interventions:

- **Aspirin:** 324 mg administered orally once.
- **Nitroglycerin:** 0.4 mg administered sublingually (SL), with the option of repeating the dose every five minutes for a maximum of three doses.
- **Morphine:** 4 mg to be administered intravenously (IVP) as needed for unrelieved chest pain.
- **Oxygen:** To maintain oxygen saturation (SpO2) levels above 92%.

MYOCARDIAL INFARCTION (MI)

Nursing Case Study #1
(Page 3)

These interventions were implemented to address the patient's myocardial infarction (heart attack) and alleviate associated symptoms, with a focus on relieving chest pain, improving oxygenation, and closely monitoring vital signs pending further diagnostic results.

Critical Thinking Check #3 *(Bloom's Taxonomy: Analysis)*
What intervention should you, as the nurse, perform right away? Why?

Critical Thinking Check #4 *(Bloom's Taxonomy: Analysis)*
What medication should be the first one administered to this patient? Why? How often?

Critical Thinking Check #5 *(Bloom's Taxonomy: Analysis)*
What is the significance of the ST-segment changes on Mr. Salazar's 12-lead EKG?

Mr. Salazar's chest pain was unrelieved after three (3) doses of sublingual nitroglycerin (NTG). Morphine 5 mg intravenous push (IVP) was administered, as well as 324 mg chewable baby aspirin. His pain was still unrelieved at this point

Mr. Salazar's cardiac enzyme results were as follows:

- **CK** 254 U/L
- **CK-MB** 10%
- **Troponin I** 3.5 ng/mL

MYOCARDIAL INFARCTION (MI)

Nursing Case Study #1
(Page 4)

Critical Thinking Check #6	*(Bloom's Taxonomy: Analysis)*
Based on the results of Mr. Salazar's labs and his response to medications, what is the next intervention you anticipate? Why?	

Mr. Salazar was taken immediately to the cath lab for a Percutaneous Coronary Intervention (PCI). The cardiologist found a 90% blockage in his left anterior descending (LAD) artery. A stent was inserted to keep the vessel open.

Critical Thinking Check #7	*(Bloom's Taxonomy: Comprehension)*
What is the purpose of Percutaneous Coronary Intervention (PCI), also known as a heart catheterization?	

Mr. Salazar tolerated the PCI well and was admitted to the cardiac telemetry unit for observation overnight. Four (4) hours after the procedure, Mr. Salazar reports no chest pain. His vital signs are now as follows:

- **BP** 128/82 mmHg SpO2 96% on 2L NC
- **HR 76** bpm and regular RR 18 bpm
- **Temp** 37.1°C

Mr. Salazar will be discharged home 24 hours after his arrival to the ED and will follow up with his cardiologist next week.

Critical Thinking Check #8	*(Bloom's Taxonomy: Application)*
What patient education topics would need to be covered with Mr. Salazar?	

MYOCARDIAL INFARCTION (MI)

Nursing Case Study #1
(Page 5)

In summary, Mr. Salazar's case highlights the urgency of recognizing and responding to myocardial infarction promptly. The application of vital signs, EKG, cardiac enzymes, and medications like aspirin, nitroglycerin, and morphine played a pivotal role in his care. Diagnostic tools like echocardiography and chest X-rays contributed to a comprehensive evaluation.

Nurses must remain vigilant and compassionate in such emergencies. This case study emphasizes the importance of adhering to best practices in the assessment, diagnosis, and management of myocardial infarction, with the ultimate goal of achieving favorable patient outcomes.

Answer Key:

💡 **Critical Thinking Check #1:**

Full set of vital signs
- Heart Rate (HR): The number of heartbeats per minute.
- Blood Pressure (BP): The force of blood against the walls of the arteries, typically measured as systolic (during heartbeats) and diastolic (between heartbeats) pressure.
- Respiratory Rate (RR): The number of breaths a patient takes per minute.
- Body Temperature (Temp): The measurement of a patient's internal body heat.
- Oxygen Saturation (SpO2): The percentage of oxygen in the blood.

Heart sounds
- Heart sounds are the noises generated by the beating heart and can be classified into two main components:
- S1: The first heart sound, often described as "lub," is caused by the
- closure of the mitral and tricuspid valves.
- S2: The second heart sound, known as "dub," results from the closure of the aortic and pulmonic valves.

MYOCARDIAL INFARCTION (MI)

Nursing Case Study #1
(Page 6)

Answer Key: Continued

- These sounds provide important diagnostic information about the condition of the heart.

Lung sounds
- Lung sounds are noises heard during the physical examination of the chest and can be categorized as: Clear- Normal, healthy lung sounds with no added sounds.
- Crackles (Rales): Discontinuous, often high-pitched sounds are heard with conditions like pneumonia or heart failure.
- Wheezes: Whistling, musical sounds often associated with conditions like asthma or chronic obstructive pulmonary disease (COPD).

Pulses
- Pulses refer to the rhythmic expansion and contraction of arteries with each heartbeat. Common pulse points for assessment include the radial artery (wrist), carotid artery (neck), and femoral artery (groin). Evaluating pulses helps assess the strength, regularity, and rate of blood flow.

Edema
- Edema is the abnormal accumulation of fluid in body tissues, leading to swelling. It can occur in various body parts and may indicate underlying conditions such as heart failure, kidney disease, or localized injury. Edema assessment involves evaluating degree of swelling and its location.

Skin condition (temperature, color, etc.)

Critical Thinking Check #2:

Oxygen
- Oxygen therapy involves administering oxygen to a patient to increase the level of oxygen in their blood. It is used to treat conditions such as respiratory distress, and hypoxia (low oxygen levels), and to support patients with breathing difficulties.

MYOCARDIAL INFARCTION (MI)

Nursing Case Study #1
(Page 7)

Answer Key: Continued

Nitroglycerin
- Nitroglycerin is a medication used to treat angina (chest pain) and to relieve symptoms of heart-related conditions. It works by relaxing and widening blood vessels, which improves blood flow to the heart, reducing chest pain.

Aspirin
- Aspirin is a common over-the-counter medication and antiplatelet drug. In the context of myocardial infarction (heart attack), it is often administered to reduce blood clot formation, potentially preventing further blockage in coronary arteries.

12-Lead EKG
- A 12-lead EKG is a diagnostic test that records the electrical activity of the heart from 12 different angles. It provides information about the heart's rhythm, rate, and any abnormalities, helping diagnose conditions like arrhythmias, heart attacks, and ischemia.

Cardiac Enzymes
- Cardiac enzymes are proteins released into the bloodstream when heart muscle cells are damaged or die, typically during a heart attack. Measuring these enzymes, such as troponin and creatine kinase-MB (CK-MB), helps confirm a heart attack diagnosis and assess its severity.

Chest X-ray
- A chest X-ray is a diagnostic imaging procedure that creates images of the chest and its internal structures, including the heart and lungs. It is used to identify issues like lung infections, heart enlargement, fluid accumulation, or fractures in the chest area.

Possibly an Echocardiogram

Critical Thinking Check #3:

- Apply oxygen – this can be done quickly and easily and can help to prevent further complications from low oxygenation.

MYOCARDIAL INFARCTION (MI)

Nursing Case Study #1
(Page 8)

Answer Key: Continued

- Oxygen helps to improve oxygenation as well as to decrease myocardial oxygen demands.
- Often it takes a few minutes or more for medications to be available from the pharmacy, so it makes sense to take care of this intervention first.
- ABC's – breathing/O2.

Critical Thinking Check #4:

- Nitroglycerin 0.4mg SL – it is a vasodilator and works on the coronary arteries. The goal is to increase blood flow to the myocardium. If this is effective, the patient merely has angina. However, if it is not effective, the patient may have a myocardial infarction.
- Aspirin should also be given, but it is to decrease platelet aggregation and reduce mortality. While it can somewhat help prevent the worsening of the blockage, it does little for the current pain experienced by the patient.
- Morphine should only be given if the nitroglycerin and aspirin do not relieve the patient's chest pain.

Critical Thinking Check #5:

- ST-segment changes on a 12-lead EKG indicate ischemia (lack of oxygen-/blood flow) or infarction (death of the muscle tissue) of the myocardium (heart muscle).
- This indicates an emergent situation. The patient's coronary arteries are blocked and need to be reopened by pharmacological (thrombolytic) or surgical (PCI) intervention.
- Time is tissue – the longer the coronary arteries stay blocked, the more of the patient's myocardium that will die. Dead heart tissue doesn't beat.

MYOCARDIAL INFARCTION (MI)

Nursing Case Study #1
(Page 9)

Answer Key: Continued

Critical Thinking Check #6:

- Mr. Salazar needs intervention. He will either receive thrombolytics or a heart catheterization (PCI).
- Based on the EKG changes, elevated Troponin level, and the fact that his symptoms are not subsiding, it's possible the patient has a significant blockage in one or more of his coronary arteries.
- It seems as though it may be an Anterior-Lateral MI, because ST elevation is occurring in I, aVL, and V2-V6.

Critical Thinking Check #7:

- A PCI serves to open up any coronary arteries that are blocked. First, they use contrast dye to determine where the blockage is, then they use a special balloon catheter to open the blocked vessels.
- If that doesn't work, they will place a cardiac stent in the vessel to keep it open.
- Blood flow will be restored to the myocardium with minimal residual damage.
- The patient should have baseline vital signs, relief of chest pain, normal oxygenation status, and absence of heart failure symptoms (above baseline).
- The patient should be able to ambulate without significant chest pain or SOB.
- The patient should be free from bleeding or hematoma at the site of catheterization (often femoral, but can also be radial or (rarely) carotid.

MYOCARDIAL INFARCTION (MI)

Nursing Case Study #1
(Page 10)

Answer Key: Continued

Critical Thinking Check #8:

- He should be taught any dietary and lifestyle changes that should be made.
- Diet – low sodium, low cholesterol, avoid sugar/soda, avoid fried/processed foods.
- Exercise – 30-45 minutes of moderate activity 5-7 days a week, unless instructed otherwise by a cardiologist. This will be determined by the patient's activity tolerance – how much can they do and still be able to breathe and be pain-free?
- Stop smoking and avoid caffeine and alcohol.
- Medication Instructions
- Nitroglycerin – take one SL tab at the onset of chest pain. If the pain does not subside after 5 minutes, call 911 and take a second dose. You can take a 3rd dose 5 minutes after the second if the pain does not subside. Do NOT take it if you have taken Viagra in the last 24 hours.
- Aspirin – take 81 mg of baby aspirin daily
- Anticoagulant – the patient may be prescribed an anticoagulant if they had a stent placed. They should be taught about bleeding risks.
- When to call the provider – CP unrelieved by nitroglycerin after 5 minutes. Syncope. Evidence of bleeding in stool or urine (if on anticoagulant). Palpitations, shortness of breath, or difficulty tolerating activities of daily living.

ACUTE KIDNEY INJURY (AKI)

Nursing Case Study #1
(Acute Kidney Injury)

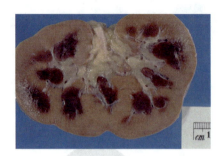

Pathophysiology:
Sudden decline in the function of the kidneys usually from decreased blood flow to the kidneys or injury to the kidney from inflammation and toxins. Acute kidney injury can be reversed if diagnosed and treated early but can progress to renal failure.

Patient:
Ms. Barkley is a thin, frail 64-year-old female presenting from a nursing home for acute abdominal pain, nausea, and vomiting x 2 days. She receives a CT scan with IV contrast. Findings show no acute bleeding, but a possible small bowel obstruction. She is admitted for bowel rest, with the following written orders from the provider:

- Continuous Telemetry
- Strict I&O measurements
- Keep SpO2 > 92%
- Keep NPO (strict)
- Hydrocodone/Acetaminophen 5-325 mg PO q6h PRN moderate to severe pain
- Ondansetron 4mg PRN nausea

She is admitted to the unit at the beginning of shift, and the UAP reports the following vital signs:

- **HR** 103
- **RR** 16
- **BP** 118/68
- **SpO2** 96%
- **Pain** 6/10

ACUTE KIDNEY INJURY (AKI)

Nursing Case Study #2
(Page 2)

***Test your knowledge by referencing the answer key at the end of this study!*

Critical Thinking Check #1 *(Bloom's Taxonomy: Apply)*
Which order would you question or request clarification for? Why?

Critical Thinking Check #2 *(Bloom's Taxonomy: Apply)*
What additional nursing assessments need to be performed?

At the end of the 12-hour shift, vital signs are as follows:

- **HR** 96 RR 22
- **BP** 147/80 SpO2 93%
- **Pain** 3/10

The nurse recognizes that the patient has not voided all day and assists the patient to the bathroom. The patient voids 200 mL dark, concentrated urine.

Critical Thinking Check #3 *(Bloom's Taxonomy: Apply)*
What nursing action(s) should be implemented at this time? Who should this information be passed on to?

Provider orders a 500 mL bolus of Normal Saline (0.9%) IV over 1 hour and a renal function panel, which is drawn promptly by the nurse. After 6 hours, Ms. Barkley still has had no further urine output. A bladder scan shows approximately 60 mL of urine in the bladder. A head-to-toe assessment now reveals crackles in Ms. Barkley's lungs and her SpO2 is 89%.

ACUTE KIDNEY INJURY (AKI)

Nursing Case Study #2
(Page 3)

The renal function panel has resulted:

- **BUN** 56 mg/dL
- **Na** 132 mg/dL
- **Cr** 3.6 mg/dL
- **Ca** 7.7 mg/dL
- **GFR** 47 mL/min/m2
- **Phos** 4.8 mg/dL
- **K** 5.5 mEq/L
- **Mg** 1.4 mg/dL

Critical Thinking Check #4	(Bloom's Taxonomy: Analyze)
What nursing action(s) should be implemented at this time?	

Critical Thinking Check #5	(Bloom's Taxonomy: Analyze)
What orders should be anticipated from the provider?	

Critical Thinking Check #6	(Bloom's Taxonomy: Analyze)
What is going on physiologically with Ms. Barkley at this time? Explain what contributed to the development of this condition	

The provider orders to give 1L bolus of Normal Saline (0.9%) over 1 hour, then 125 mL/hr of Normal Saline continuously. The provider also orders a one-time dose of 40 mg Furosemide IV push and to re-check the Renal Function Panel in 6 hours. Ms. Barkley diuresis approximately 600 mL in 2

ACUTE KIDNEY INJURY (AKI)

Nursing Case Study #2
(Page 4)

and her lungs now sound clear to auscultation. Over the next two days, Ms. Barkley's hourly urine output begins to improve and her BUN, Creatinine, and GFR return to normal ranges. Her small bowel obstruction resolves on its own and she is able to begin taking PO food and fluids.

Critical Thinking Check #3	(Bloom's Taxonomy: Apply)
What nursing action(s) should be implemented at this time? Who should this information be passed on to?	

Answer Key:

Critical Thinking Check #1:

- The Ondansetron order is incomplete. There is no route or frequency ordered.

Critical Thinking Check #2

- The Ondansetron order is incomplete. There is no route or frequency ordered
- Assess abdomen – inspect, auscultate, palpate and percuss. Assess for tenderness over specific areas, feel for masses, and look for guarding.
- Listen to heart and lung sounds to ensure no cardiac involvement
- Assess pain with a detailed pain assessment so that pain can be treated appropriately
- Assess skin – the patient has had nausea/vomiting for 2 days, there may be some dehydration – check for tenting.

ACUTE KIDNEY INJURY (AKI)

Nursing Case Study #2
(Page 5)

Answer Key: Continued

💡 Critical Thinking Check #3:

- Document the output, notify the provider of the decreased urine output. This information needs to be passed onto the oncoming nurse so that he or she can closely monitor the patient's urine output.

💡 Critical Thinking Check #4

- Administer O2 2 lpm via nasal cannula (to keep sats > 92%)
- Notify the provider of lab results, especially BUN/Cr, GFR, and Potassium – as these indicate there is kidney involvement.

💡 Critical Thinking Check #5

- The patient may need more fluids, she's been vomiting for 2 days and NPO for another 12 hours with no IV fluids.
- The patient may require diuretics to remove the excess fluid from her lungs and to determine the level of function of her kidneys

💡 Critical Thinking Check #6

- Ms. Barkley seems to have developed an acute kidney injury or acute kidney failure. The likely contributors are the severe dehydration coupled with the IV contrast and 12+ hours of being NPO and having no IV fluids. This caused a low-flow state to the kidneys (pre-renal) as well as possible damage to the kidneys themselves because of the contrast (intrarenal).

ACUTE KIDNEY INJURY (AKI)

Nursing Case Study #2
(Page 6)

Answer Key: Continued

💡 **Critical Thinking Check #7:**

- The best option would have been to give Ms. Barkley IV fluids before and after her contrast scan, and to make sure she had maintenance IV fluids infusing while she was NPO. Depending on the patient's kidney function, it isn't always preventable, but in this case, it seems there was more that could have been done.

CIRRHOSIS

📄 **Nursing Case Study #3 (Cirrhosis)**

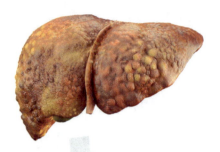

Pathophysiology:
Cirrhosis is late stage liver fibrosis. It causes the normal blood flow to slow through the liver. This increases the pressure in the vein that carries blood from the intestines and spleen to the liver. This increased pressure in the portal vein will cause fluid to back up and accumulate in the legs and abdomen.

Patient:
Mr. Garcia is a 43-year-old male who presented to the ED complaining of nausea and vomiting x 3 days. The nurse notes a large, distended abdomen and yellowing of the patient's skin and eyes. The patient reports a history of alcoholic cirrhosis.

***Test your knowledge by referencing the answer key at the end of this study!

Critical Thinking Check #1 (Bloom's Taxonomy: Application)
What initial nursing assessments should be performed?

Critical Thinking Check #2 (Bloom's Taxonomy: Analysis)
What diagnostic testing do you anticipate for Mr. Garcia?

Mr. Garcia's vitals are stable, BP 100/58, bowel sounds are active but distant, and the nurse notes a positive fluid wave test on his abdomen. The patient denies itching but is constantly scratching at his chest. He is oriented to person only and his brother at the bedside reports he hasn't been himself today. He keeps trying to get out of bed.

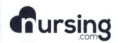

NURSING.com - "Tools and Confidence to Succeed in Nursing School."
©2023 TazKai LLC | NURSING.com - Reproduction Strictly Prohibited
Disclaimer information at NURSING.com

CIRRHOSIS

Nursing Case Study #3
(Page 2)

Critical Thinking Check #3	*(Bloom's Taxonomy: Analysis)*

Which finding is most concerning and needs to be reported to the provider? Why?

Critical Thinking Check #4	*(Bloom's Taxonomy: Analysis)*

What further diagnostic and lab tests should be ordered to determine Mr. Garcia's priority problems?

The provider places orders for the following:

- Keep SpO2 > 92%
- Keep HOB > 30 degrees
- Insert 2 large bore PIV's
- 500 mL NS IV bolus STAT
- 100 mL/hr NS IV continuous infusion
- Hydrocodone/Acetaminophen 5-500 mg 1-2 tabs q4h PRN moderate to severe pain
- Diphenhydramine 25 mg PO q8h PRN itching
- Ondansetron 4 mg IV q6h PRN nausea
- Lactulose 20 mg PO q6h

Mr. Garcia's LFT's and Ammonia levels are elevated. He is extremely confused and agitated and appears somewhat short of breath. The patient's current vital signs are as follows:

- **HR** 82 RR 22
- **BP** 94/56 SpO2 93%
- **Temp** 98.9°F

CIRRHOSIS

Nursing Case Study #3
(Page 3)

Critical Thinking Check #5   (Bloom's Taxonomy: Analysis)

Which order should be implemented first? Why?

Critical Thinking Check #6   (Bloom's Taxonomy: Analysis)

Which order should be questioned? Why?

The order is changed to Fentanyl 25 mcg IV q4h PRN moderate to severe pain. The provider notes somewhat shallow breathing and severe ascites and requests for you to set up for paracentesis. At this time, you express your concern that the patient is extremely confused and agitated and trying to get out of bed. You do not feel that he will be still enough for the procedure. The provider agrees and plans to postpone the paracentesis for now, but orders for you to report any signs of respiratory depression or hypoxia.

Critical Thinking Check #7   (Bloom's Taxonomy: Analysis)

Why is Mr. Garcia so confused and agitated?

Critical Thinking Check #8   (Bloom's Taxonomy: Analysis)

What is the rationale for performing a paracentesis for Mr. Garcia?

After 6 doses of lactulose, Mr. Garcia is much more calm and cooperative. He is oriented times 2-3 most times. The provider performs the paracentesis and is able to remove 1.5 L of fluid. The patient's shortness of breath is

CIRRHOSIS

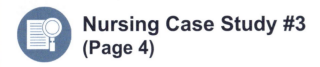

Nursing Case Study #3
(Page 4)

relieved, and his breathing is less shallow. Ultrasound of the liver showed severe scarring on the liver. Mr. Garcia's condition continues to improve, and the plan is to discharge him home tomorrow.

Critical Thinking Check #9	*(Bloom's Taxonomy: Application)*
What discharge teaching should be included for Mr. Garcia, including nutrition?	

Answer Key:

💡 **Critical Thinking Check #1:**

- Full abdominal assessment, including assessing for ascites
- Heart and lung sounds
- Skin assessment – color, turgor, etc.
- Full set of vital signs
- Neurological assessment

💡 **Critical Thinking Check #2**

- LFT's, CBC, BMP

💡 **Critical Thinking Check #3**

- Confusion, disorientation – this could indicate hepatic encephalopathy, which could lead to seizures and death if left untreated

💡 **Critical Thinking Check #4**

- Abdominal X-ray and/or Abdominal ultrasound to visualize liver and whether the distended abdomen is related to ascites or other sources

CIRRHOSIS

Nursing Case Study #3
(Page 5)

Answer Key: Continued

- Ammonia level to determine if hepatic encephalopathy is the source of Mr. Garcia's altered mental status.

💡 Critical Thinking Check #5:

- Insert two large-bore IV's. The patient requires IV fluids and has other IV meds ordered and will likely need labs drawn. This needs to be a priority.
- You could also say elevate the HOB to 30 degrees or higher, if there was indication that he was lying flat
- His SpO2 is >92%, so no intervention is required there.
- Lactulose should be the next priority intervention – to get the ammonia levels down – but it may take a bit for pharmacy to profile it, send it to the unit, etc.

💡 Critical Thinking Check #6

- Hydrocodone/Acetaminophen – Acetaminophen can be toxic for patients with liver disease. The way this order is written, this patient could receive anywhere from 3 g – 6 g of Acetaminophen in a 24-hour period. The max for a healthy person is 4 g, but for liver patients, it is 2 g max.
- Either the dose and frequency should be lowered significantly, or the medication should be changed altogether

💡 Critical Thinking Check #7

- His ammonia levels are elevated due to his liver failure – this causes hepatic encephalopathy – damage to the brain cells
- This causes altered mental status, agitation, confusion, and can eventually lead to seizures and death if left untreated

CIRRHOSIS

Nursing Case Study #3
(Page 6)

Answer Key: Continued

Critical Thinking Check #8:

- The excess fluid in Mr. Garcia's belly is compressing his thoracic cavity, causing him to feel short of breath and to only take shallow breaths. Draining this fluid will not only relieve some discomfort, but it can also help improve Mr. Garcia's breathing

Critical Thinking Check #9:

- Mr. Garcia should not be eating a high protein diet as this can contribute to the increased ammonia levels and development of hepatic encephalopathy.
- Mr. Garcia should avoid drinking alcohol at all times
- Medication instructions for any new or changed medications
- Especially the importance of taking Lactulose regularly as ordered
- Signs to report to the provider of exacerbation or encephalopathy

COPD

**Nursing Case Study #4
COPD-
(Chronic Obstructive Pulmonary Disease))**

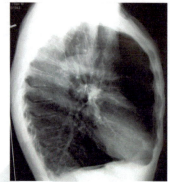

Pathophysiology:
COPD stands for chronic obstructive pulmonary disease and includes emphysema, chronic bronchitis, and asthma. In a healthy individual air sacs are elastic and expand as the person inhales. When the healthy individual exhales the air sacs will then deflate. In COPD the air sacs are not as stretchy and are damaged with inflammation and thickness. The airways become obstructed with mucus. These factors make breathing and gas exchange a challenge.

Patient:
Mr. Whaley is a 65-year-old man with a history of COPD who presents to his primary care provider's (PCP) office complaining of a productive cough off and on for 2 years and shortness of breath for the last 3 days. He reports that he has had several chest colds in the last few years, but this time it won't go away. His wife says he has been feverish for a few days, but doesn't have a specific temperature to report. He reports smoking a pack of

***Test your knowledge by referencing the answer key at the end of this study!*

Critical Thinking Check #1 (Bloom's Taxonomy: Application)
What nursing assessments should be performed at this time for Mr. Whaley?

Upon further assessment, Mr. Whaley has crackles throughout the lower lobes of his lungs, with occasional expiratory wheezes throughout the lung fields. His vital signs are as follows:

- **BP** 142/86 mmHg **HR** 102 bpm

COPD

Nursing Case Study #4
(Page 2)

- **RR** 32 bpm Temp 38.8°C
- **SpO2** 86% on room air

The nurse locates a portable oxygen tank and places the patient on 2 lpm oxygen via nasal cannula. Based on these findings, Mr. Whaley's PCP decides to call an ambulance to send Mr. Whaley to the Emergency Department (ED). While waiting for the ambulance, the nurse repeats the SpO2 and finds Mr. Whaley's SpO2 is only 89%. She increases his oxygen to 4 lpm, rechecks and notes an SpO2 of 95%. The ambulance crew arrives, the nurse reports to them that the patient was short of breath and hypoxic, but sats are now 95% and he is resting. Per EMS, he is alert and oriented x 3.

Critical Thinking Check #2 *(Bloom's Taxonomy: Analysis)*
What is going on with Mr. Whaley, physiologically?

Critical Thinking Check #3 *(Bloom's Taxonomy: Analysis)*
What would you have done differently? Why?

Upon arrival to the ED, the RN finds Mr. Whaley is somnolent and difficult to arouse. He takes a set of vital signs and finds the following:

- **BP** 138/78 mmHg **HR** 96 bpm
- **RR** 16 bpm Temp 38.4°C
- **SpO2** 96% on 4 lpm nasal cannula

COPD

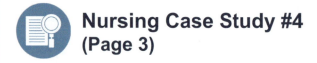

Nursing Case Study #4
(Page 3)

Critical Thinking Check #4	(Bloom's Taxonomy: Analysis)
What is the possible cause of Mr. Whaley's somnolence?	

Critical Thinking Check #5	(Bloom's Taxonomy: Analysis)
What orders do you expect from the ED provider?	

The provider writes the following orders:

- Keep sats 88-92%
- CXR
- Labs: ABG, CBC, BMP
- Insert peripheral IV
- Albuterol nebulizer 2.5mg
- Budesonide-formoterol 160/4.5 mcg

The nurse immediately removes the supplemental oxygen from Mr. Whaley and attempts to stimulate him awake. Mr. Whaley is still quite drowsy, but is able to awake long enough to state his full name. The nurse inserts a peripheral IV and draws the CBC and BMP, while the Respiratory Therapist (RT) draws an arterial blood gas (ABG). Blood gas results are as follows:

- **pH** 7.30
- **pCO2** 58 mmHg
- **HCO3**– 30 mEq/L
- **pO2** 50 mmHg
- **SaO2** 92%

COPD

Nursing Case Study #4
(Page 4)

Critical Thinking Check #6	(Bloom's Taxonomy: Application)
Interpret the ABG. Explain.	

Critical Thinking Check #7	(Bloom's Taxonomy: Analysis)
Which medication should be administered first? Why?	

Mr. Whaley's condition improves after a bronchodilator and corticosteroid breathing treatment. His SpO2 remains 90% on room air and his shortness of breath has significantly decreased. He is still running a fever of 38.3°C. The ED provider orders broad spectrum antibiotics for a likely pneumonia, which may have caused this COPD exacerbation. The provider also orders two inhalers for Mr. Whaley, one bronchodilator and one corticosteroid. Satisfied with his quick improvement, the provider decides it is safe for Mr. Whaley to recover at home with proper instructions for his medications and follow up from his PCP.

Critical Thinking Check #8	(Bloom's Taxonomy: Application)
What are priority discharge teaching topics for Mr. Whaley?	

Answer Key:

Critical Thinking Check #1:

- Full set of vital signs, including SpO2
- Heart and Lung sounds

COPD

Nursing Case Study #4
(Page 5)

Answer Key: Continued

- Gather any further details of illness or medical history, including allergies

💡 Critical Thinking Check #2:

- Mr. Whaley may have a lung infection, as evidenced by his fever and productive cough. This is causing a COPD exacerbation. COPD makes gas exchange difficult, which is why his SpO2 levels are low.

💡 Critical Thinking Check #3

- Because of his COPD, Mr. Whaley should not have been placed on more than 2 lpm of supplemental O2 because it would decrease his respiratory drive and lead to CO2 toxicity.
- When Mr. Whaley's sats didn't improve, should have notified provider before adding more supplemental oxygen

💡 Critical Thinking Check #4

- His COPD makes gas exchange difficult, therefore he retains CO2. This means his respiratory drive to breathe is low O2 instead of high CO2. When the nurse gave too much supplemental oxygen, Mr. Whaley lost some of his respiratory drive. This is why his respiratory rate is so low.
- This can lead to CO2 toxicity, which presents as a decreased LOC and decreased respiratory rate, and can lead to the patient not protecting their airway and going into respiratory arrest

💡 Critical Thinking Check #5

- To remove the supplemental oxygen and only keep SpO2 between 88-92% to avoid over-oxygenating and CO2 toxicity

COPD

Nursing Case Study #4
(Page 6)

Answer Key: Continued

- Chest X-ray
- Blood Cultures, Sputum Cultures, CBC, BMP, ABG
- Bronchodilators, Corticosteroids, Breathing treatments from Respiratory Therapy

Critical Thinking Check #6:

- This is respiratory acidosis with partial compensation
- The ABG also shows hypoxemia
- Mr. Whaley retains CO_2 chronically and his kidneys have tried to compensate (as evidenced by the HCO_3^- of 30 mEq/L). They weren't able to fully compensate, though, so his pH is still acidic because of the high CO_2

Critical Thinking Check #7:

- Albuterol – because it is a bronchodilator and should always be administered before corticosteroids

Critical Thinking Check #8:

- Mr. Whaley NEEDS to stop smoking!!!
- Proper use of inhalers, new medication instructions
- Reporting s/s respiratory infection to PCP sooner

PNEUMONIA

Nursing Case Study #5
(Pneumonia)

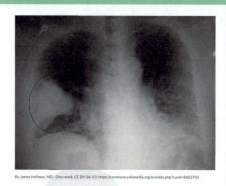

Pathophysiology:

Pneumonia is an inflammatory response. This can be caused by an infection or things like aspiration where fluid gets into the lungs, which causes the alveoli to fill with fluid or pus. When the alveoli are filled with fluid or pus then proper gas exchange does not occur as well.

Patient:

Charles is a 72-year-old male patient admitted via the emergency department to the medical surgical floor at 2220 with a diagnosis of community acquired pneumonia (CAP). He arrives in the room via stretcher with oxygen (O2) via nasal cannula (NC) and is able to transfer to the bed with minimal assistance. He does get short of breath (SOB) with exertion.

*** Test your knowledge by referencing the answer key at the end of this study!*

Critical Thinking Check #1	*(Bloom's Taxonomy: Analyze)*
What assessment findings does the nurse expect for this patient? Should there be a particular focus to the assessment?	

Critical Thinking Check #2	*(Bloom's Taxonomy: Analyze)*
Are there any ER results the nurse should ask about during the bedside report?	

Critical Thinking Check #3	*(Bloom's Taxonomy: Evaluate)*
What orders does the nurse expect the admitting provider to give?	

NURSING.com - "Tools and Confidence to Succeed in Nursing School."
©2023 TazKai LLC | NURSING.com - Reproduction Strictly Prohibited
Disclaimer information at NURSING.com

PNEUMONIA

**Nursing Case Study #5
(Page 2)**

After screening and assessing the patient, the nurse has the following data:

Patient AA&Ox4. SOB noted with speaking and after he moves around. IV 20g noted in the left arm. Productive cough with moderate sputum production occasionally. Lung sounds in all fields indicate crackles; no barrel chest noted. Skin is warm and dry. He voids per urinal no assistance needed. Verbalizes understanding of call light use.

- **BP** 120/60 SpO2 93% on NC 2L
- **HR** 100 bpm and regular Ht 172 cm
- **RR** 18 bpm Wt 60 kg
- **Temp** 38.3°C

CXR – posteroanterior and lateral chest radiographs obtained (two view). Radiographic findings consistent with the diagnosis of CAP including minor lobar consolidations, moderate interstitial infiltrates.

- **CBC** (abnormal/significant only listed, if NOT listed then the value falls within expected limits or is not significant for this patient), for reference see nursing.com Lab Value cheat sheet:
- **WBC** 15,000 cells/mcL
- **Bands** 10%
- **Neutrophils** 60%
- **Eosinophils** 1%
- **Basophils** 1%
- **Lymphocytes** 20%

Critical Thinking Check #4	*(Bloom's Taxonomy: Evaluate)*
Prioritize the top nursing interventions.	

PNEUMONIA

Nursing Case Study #5
(Page 3)

Critical Thinking Check #5 (Bloom's Taxonomy: Evaluate)

What should the nurse be on the lookout for as the shift progresses? What warrants a call to the provider?

Critical Thinking Check #6 (Bloom's Taxonomy: Evaluate)

Are there other orders the nurse might anticipate and/or suggest?

Critical Thinking Check #7 (Bloom's Taxonomy: Analyze)

Are there past medical history concerns specific to this patient and his background that may aid in the plan of care?

ABG values:

- **pH** 7.30
- **PaCO2** 50 mmHg
- **HCO3-** 23 mEq/L
- **PaO2** 88 mmHg

Critical Thinking Check #8 (Bloom's Taxonomy: Analyze)

What does this ABG indicate? How do you know? What may have caused this value? What can you do?

PNEUMONIA

Nursing Case Study #5
(Page 4)

The nurse gets the CNA to assist and repositions Charles in his hospital bed and he now sits straight but comfortably up in bed with pillows to bolster him. A yankauer at the bedside that he can use for a productive cough allows him to clear his airway after a brief teaching session. He had been frequently removing his NC due to ear discomfort, so RT brought padding for the tubing and Charles reports improved comfort. RT and the nurse teach him about "turn, cough, deep breath" aka TCDB.

After sleeping on and off through the shift, Charles is able to consume approximately 75% of his breakfast. He can properly demonstrate use of his IS and TCDB techniques. His NC remains in place with the padding on ears and his O2 sat is 95% on 2 L. He has two functioning IVs, one in each arm. Physician rounds and advises to continue plan of care including medication regimen based on test results after he and nurse discuss patient during rounds with the clinical pharmacist.

Critical Thinking Check #9	(Bloom's Taxonomy: Apply)
Describe examples of interdisciplinary team collaboration that may be useful in this patient's care.	

Answer Key:

Critical Thinking Check #1:

- The Ondansetron order is incomplete. There is no route or frequency ordered.

Critical Thinking Check #2:

- The Ondansetron order is incomplete. No route or frequency ordered

PNEUMONIA

Nursing Case Study #5
(Page 5)

Answer Key: Continued

- Assess abdomen – inspect, auscultate, palpate and percuss. Assess for tenderness over specific areas, feel for masses, and look for guarding.
- Listen to heart and lung sounds to ensure no cardiac involvement
- Assess pain with a detailed pain assessment so that pain can be treated appropriately
- Assess skin – the patient has had nausea/vomiting for 2 days, there may be some dehydration – check for tenting.

Critical Thinking Check #3

- Document the output, notify the provider of the decreased urine output. This information needs to be passed onto the oncoming nurse so that he or she can closely monitor the patient's urine output.

Critical Thinking Check #4

- Administer O2 2 lpm via nasal cannula (to keep sats > 92%)
- Notify the provider of lab results, especially BUN/Cr, GFR, and Potassium – as these indicate there is kidney involvement.

Critical Thinking Check #5

- The patient may need more fluids, she's been vomiting for 2 days and NPO for another 12 hours with no IV fluids.
- The patient may require diuretics to remove the excess fluid from her lungs and to determine the level of function of her kidneys

Critical Thinking Check #6

- Ms. Barkley seems to have developed an acute kidney injury or acute kidney failure. The likely contributors are the severe dehydration coupled-

PNEUMONIA

Nursing Case Study #5
(Page 6)

Answer Key: Continued

- with the IV contrast and 12+ hours of being NPO and having no IV fluids. This caused a low-flow state to the kidneys (pre-renal) as well as possible damage to the kidneys themselves because of the contrast (intrarenal).

Critical Thinking Check #7:

- The best option would have been to give Ms. Barkley IV fluids before and after her contrast scan, and to make sure she had maintenance IV fluids infusing while she was NPO. Depending on the patient's kidney function, it isn't always preventable, but in this case, it seems there was more that could have been done.

STROKE

Nursing Case Study #6 (Stroke)

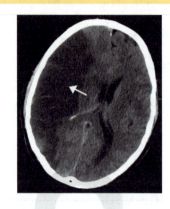

By INFARCT.jpg: Lucien Monfilsderivative work: Suraj - INFARCT.jpg, CC BY-SA 3.0, https://commons.wikimedia.org/w/index.php?curid=16444670

Pathophysiology:
A stroke is essentially a neurological deficit caused by decreased blood flow to a portion of the brain. They will be classified as either hemorrhagic or ischemic. An ischemic stroke is the result of an obstruction of blood flow within a blood vessel. A hemorrhagic stroke is when a weakened blood vessel ruptures and blood spills into the brain where it shouldn't be. Both of these can cause edema and cellular death. Lack of blood flow for greater than 10 minutes can cause irreversible damage.

Patient:
Mrs. Blossom is a 57-year-old female who presented to the Emergency Room with new onset Atrial Fibrillation with Rapid Ventricular Response (RVR). She is admitted to the cardiac telemetry unit after being converted to normal sinus rhythm with a calcium channel blocker (diltiazem). When you enter the room to assess Mrs. Blossom, her daughter looks at you concerned and says "mom's acting kinda funny."

***Test your knowledge by referencing the answer key at the end of this study!**

Critical Thinking Check #1	(Bloom's Taxonomy: Application)
What nursing assessments should be completed at this time?	

You assess Mrs. Blossom to find she has a left sided facial droop, slurred speech, and is unable to hold her left arm up for more than 3 seconds.

STROKE

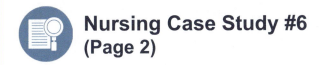

Nursing Case Study #6
(Page 2)

Critical Thinking Check #2 *(Bloom's Taxonomy: Analysis)*
What is/are your priority nursing action(s) at this time?

Critical Thinking Check #3 *(Bloom's Taxonomy: Analysis)*
What may be occurring in Mrs. Blossom?

You call a Code Stroke and notify the charge nurse for help. You obtain suction to have at bedside just in case. The neurologist arrives at bedside within 7 minutes to assess Mrs. Blossom. He notes her NIH Stroke Scale score is 32. He orders a STAT CT scan, which shows there is no obvious bleed in the brain.

Critical Thinking Check #4 *(Bloom's Taxonomy: Analysis)*
What are the possible interventions for Mrs. Blossom at this time?

Critical Thinking Check #5 *(Bloom's Taxonomy: Comprehension)*
What are the contraindications for thrombolytics like tPA (alteplase)?

You administer tPA per protocol, initiate q15min vital signs and neuro checks. You stay with the patient to continue to monitor her symptoms.

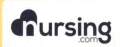

STROKE

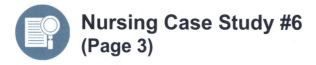

Nursing Case Study #6
(Page 3)

Critical Thinking Check #6 (Bloom's Taxonomy: Comprehension)
What are possible complications of tPA administration? What should you monitor for?

After 2 hours, Mrs. Blossom is showing signs of improvement. She is able to speak more clearly, though with a slight slur. She is still slightly weak on the left side, but is able to hold her arm up for 10 seconds now. Her NIHSS is now 6. Mrs. Blossom's daughter asks you why this happened.

Critical Thinking Check #7 (Bloom's Taxonomy: Analysis)
What would you explain has happened to Mrs. Blossom physiologically?

Two days later, Mrs. Blossom has recovered fully. She will be discharged today on Clopidogrel and Aspirin, plus a calcium channel blocker, with a follow up appointment in 1 week to see the neurologist.

Critical Thinking Check #8 (Bloom's Taxonomy: Application)
What education topics should be included in the discharge teaching for Mrs. Blossom and her family?

Answer Key:

 Critical Thinking Check #1:

- Full set of vital signs (Temp, HR, BP, RR, SpO2)
- Should probably get a 12-lead EKG
- Assess symptoms using PQRST or OLDCARTS

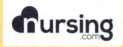

STROKE

Nursing Case Study #6
(Page 4)

Answer Key: Continued

Critical Thinking Check #2:

- Call a Code Stroke (or whatever the equivalent is at your facility) to initiate response of the neurologist or Stroke team.
- Notify the charge nurse to help you obtain emergency equipment if you don't already have it at the bedside to be prepared in case of emergency

Critical Thinking Check #3:

- She may be having a stroke

Critical Thinking Check #4:

- Since there is no bleed evident on scan, Mrs. Blossom would qualify for a thrombolytic like tPA (alteplase) or for surgical intervention, as long as there are no contraindications

Critical Thinking Check #5:

- Recent surgery, current or recent GI bleed within the last 3 months, excessive hypertension, evidence of cerebral hemorrhage

Critical Thinking Check #6:

- Bleeding, especially into the brain or a GI bleed
- She may bruise easily or bleed from IV sites or her gums
- Monitor for s/s bleeding or worsening stroke symptoms, which may indicate a hemorrhagic stroke has developed.

Critical Thinking Check #7:

STROKE

Nursing Case Study #6 (Page 5)

Answer Key: Continued

- Because of her new onset atrial fibrillation, the blood was likely pooling in her atria because they were just quivering and not contracting. When blood pools, it clots. When she was converted back into a normal rhythm and her atria began contracting again, that likely dislodged a clot, which went to her brain.
- The clot in her brain caused brain tissue to die → ischemic stroke.

Critical Thinking Check #8

- Anticoagulant therapy is imperative to prevent further clots from forming within Mrs. Blossom's atria if she stays in Atrial Fibrillation.
- They should be taught the signs of a stroke (FAST) and call 911 if they notice them.
- They should be taught signs of Atrial Fibrillation with RVR and be sure to go to the hospital if this occurs – the patient is at higher risk for stroke.
- Medication instructions for calcium channel blockers and anticoagulants.

SEIZURES

**Nursing Case Study #7
(Seizures)**

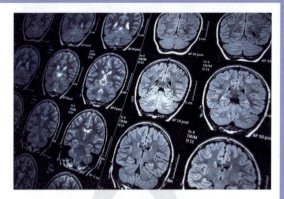

Pathophysiology:
Seizures are a very complex neurological issue. Here is the definition from Medscape of a seizure: "a seizure results when a sudden imbalance occurs between the excitatory and inhibitory forces within the network of cortical neurons in favor of a sudden-onset net excitation" (source). Basically, abnormal electrical discharges are occurring in the brain. There are different kinds of seizures (epileptic, focal-onset, general-onset).

Patient:
Ms. Cerulean is a 22 year old female admitted via EMS after a seizure witnessed by family members about 20 minutes ago. She has an IV in place.

*** Test your knowledge by referencing the answer key at the end of this study!*

Critical Thinking Check #1   *(Bloom's Taxonomy: Application)*
What initial nursing assessments need to be performed for Mr. Cerulean?

Upon assessment, Ms. Cerulean is lethargic, localizes to pain, but does not follow commands. She is diaphoretic, and her vitals are stable.

Critical Thinking Check #2   *(Bloom's Taxonomy: Analysis)*
Why is the patient experiencing a decreased level of consciousness at this time?

SEIZURES

Nursing Case Study #7
(Page 2)

Critical Thinking Check #3 *(Bloom's Taxonomy: Analysis)*

Suddenly, the patient begins jerking. Her muscles are cycling back and forth between tight contractions and rhythmic jerking. What is this called?

Critical Thinking Check #4 *(Bloom's Taxonomy: Analysis)*

What is/are your priority nursing action(s) at this time?

Critical Thinking Check #5 *(Bloom's Taxonomy: Analysis)*

What medication(s) would you expect to give to Ms. Cerulean?

Per provider orders, you administer 2mg Ativan IV Push twice in 10 minutes. Ms. Cerulean continues to seize without ceasing. The provider determines that she needs to be intubated for airway protection. Per orders, you administer a loading dose of levetiracetam and fosphenytoin and the EEG technician is on the way to place the EEG electrodes.

Critical Thinking Check #6 *(Bloom's Taxonomy: Comprehension)*

What is the name of the condition Ms. Cerulean is in now?

Critical Thinking Check #7 *(Bloom's Taxonomy: Comprehension)*

What is the purpose of the EEG?

SEIZURES

Nursing Case Study #7
(Page 3)

Ms. Cerulean is placed on a phenobarbital IV drip and additional doses of levetiracetam and fosphenytoin are administered q6h per provider orders. After 20 hours, the EEG finally begins to show decreased seizure activity.

Critical Thinking Check #8 *(Bloom's Taxonomy: Comprehension)*

What are the risks of a prolonged seizure?

Critical Thinking Check #9 *(Bloom's Taxonomy: Application)*

What education topics should be included in discharge teaching for Ms. Cerulean and her family?

Answer Key:

Critical Thinking Check #1:

- Full set of Vital Signs
- Neuro check with LOC and pupillary assessment

Critical Thinking Check #2:

- She is in a postictal state, a state of low level of consciousness that occurs after a generalized seizure for 10-30 minutes.

Critical Thinking Check #3:

- She is in a postictal state, a state of low level of consciousness that occurs after a generalized seizure for 10-30 minutes.

SEIZURES

 Nursing Case Study #7
(Page 4)

Answer Key: Continued

💡 **Critical Thinking Check #4:**

Keep the patient safe
- Turn to side
- Nothing in her mouth
- suction available if needed
- Monitor SpO2 and apply oxygen as needed
- Do not restrain
- Pad side rails to prevent injury

💡 **Critical Thinking Check #5:**

- Benzodiazepines – Ativan IV or Valium PR
- Barbiturates – Phenobarbital
- Antiepileptic drugs
- Levetiracetam, fosphenytoin, phenytoin (loading dose + maintenance dose)

💡 **Critical Thinking Check #6:**

- Because her seizures have not stopped for > 10 minutes, she is now considered to be in status epilepticus

💡 **Critical Thinking Check #7:**

- To measure brain activity to determine the severity of the seizure. It can also sometimes pinpoint where the seizure is originating
- It can also indicate whether or not seizures are still occurring, even after phenobarbital or a paralytic medication is administered.
- They should have a seizure action plan and know how to keep her safe in the event of a seizure. This includes knowing how to administer medications-
-

SEIZURES

Nursing Case Study #7
(Page 5)

Answer Key: Continued

- and when to call 911: seizure lasting longer than 5 minutes, cyanosis or apnea, or back-to-back seizures.

Critical Thinking Check #8

- Prolonged seizures can cause damage to neurons in the brain, leaving long term neurological deficits.
- Because of possible airway compromise, prolonged seizures can also lead to hypoxia, which also can cause brain damage and leave neurological deficits
- Three days later, Ms. Cerulean is awake and able to be extubated. She doesn't appear to have any neurological deficits at this time and is able to ambulate safely in the halls. She will likely be discharged home in the morning.

Critical Thinking Check #9

- Importance of compliance with antiepileptic drugs to prevent breakthrough seizures.

DIABETES MELLITUS (DM)

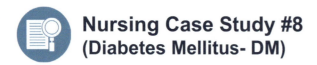

Nursing Case Study #8
(Diabetes Mellitus- DM)

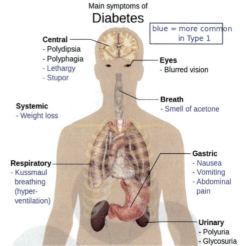

Pathophysiology:

Diabetes: Type 1 occurs when there is an autoimmune (the body attacks the pancreas) response. The beta cells are attacked and can no longer produce and secrete insulin. Insulin is necessary to take sugar from the blood to the cells for energy. Without insulin delivery sugar to the cells, hyperglycemia (high blood sugar) occurs.

Type II DM usually occurs because of genetics and or environmental factors. In type II the pancreas either does not secrete enough insulin or has difficulty with insulin action and insulin resistance occurs in the cells. Hyperglycemia occurs because the cells are resistant to insulin or because there is not adequate insulin production/secretion. When the body can not sufficiently move sugar from the blood to the cells, blood sugars rise and hyperglycemia occurs.

Patient:

Miss Matthews is a 16-year-old female who is brought to the emergency department after collapsing at school. She is currently alert, but pale and weak. A blood glucose performed by the paramedics read meter Max or high.

*** Test your knowledge by referencing the answer key at the end of this study!*

Critical Thinking Check #1   *(Bloom's Taxonomy: Application)*
What additional nursing assessments should be performed at this time?

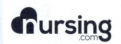

DIABETES MELLITUS (DM)

Nursing Case Study #8
(Page 2)

Critical Thinking Check #2   *(Bloom's Taxonomy: Application)*
What history questions would you like to ask of the patient and/or her parents?

Upon further questioning, the parents report that their daughter has been weak a lot lately. Miss Matthews reports but she's always hot and exhausted. She reports a 10-pound weight loss over the last 2 months despite eating all the time and agrees that she has been thirsty and peeing a lot.

Critical Thinking Check #3   *(Bloom's Taxonomy: Analysis)*
What diagnostic tests should be run for Miss Matthews?

A serum glucose revealed that Miss Matthews' blood glucose is 523 mg/dL, and her urine was positive for ketones. The provider explains that she is likely a diabetic. Her parents are shocked as she has always been a healthy and athletic child. The parents ask the nurse "How can she be diabetic when she is so skinny and exercises all of the time?"

Critical Thinking Check #4   *(Bloom's Taxonomy: Comprehension)*
What is an appropriate response by the nurse?

Critical Thinking Check #5   *(Bloom's Taxonomy: Analysis)*
What treatments do you expect to be ordered for Miss Matthews at this time?

Miss Matthews is treated for diabetic ketoacidosis over the next 2 days and is now feeling much better. The diabetic nurse educator comes by to teach Miss

DIABETES MELLITUS (DM)

Nursing Case Study #8
(Page 3)

Matthews how to self-administer SubQ insulin using an insulin pen. Miss Matthews says "I can't stand needles, isn't there a pill I can take instead?"

Critical Thinking Check #6 *(Bloom's Taxonomy: Comprehension)*
What is the most appropriate response by the nurse?

Critical Thinking Check #7 *(Bloom's Taxonomy: Comprehension)*
What options does Miss Matthews have for insulin administration?

Miss Matthews is able to demonstrate proper technique for glucose monitoring and self-administration of insulin with the insulin pen. Her blood glucose levels are stable between 140 and 180 mg/dL, and the provider has said that she could go home today.

Critical Thinking Check #8 *(Bloom's Taxonomy: Application)*
In addition to the insulin education, she has already received, what other education topics should be included in discharge teaching for Miss Matthews?

Answer Key:

Critical Thinking Check #1:

- POC glucose
- Heart and lung sounds and respiratory effort – ensure she is protecting her airway
- Assess skin and mucous membranes
- Level of consciousness and orientation

DIABETES MELLITUS (DM)

Nursing Case Study #8
(Page 4)

Answer Key: Continued

Critical Thinking Check #2:

- Has she been excessively thirsty or hungry lately
- Has she been urinating a lot
- Has she lost weight unintentionally?
- Is there a history of diabetes in the family?
- Has she been told previously that she has diabetes?
- Does she take any medications on a daily basis?

Critical Thinking Check #3:

- Serum glucose level
- BMP – electrolytes, anion gap, etc.
- Hgb A1c
- ABG to assess for acidosis
- Urine ketones

Critical Thinking Check #4:

- Your daughter has Type 1 diabetes, which means that she has an autoimmune disorder that attacks the cells in her pancreas that make insulin. Type 1 diabetes typically has nothing to do with diet and lifestyle and usually has more to do with genetics.
- Your daughter's healthy lifestyle will continue to help her control her blood sugar levels, but unfortunately, there is no cure for type 1 diabetes at this time.

Critical Thinking Check #5:

- Miss Matthews will need intensive insulin therapy and IV fluids to counteract the ketoacidosis and bring her blood sugars down.

DIABETES MELLITUS (DM)

Nursing Case Study #8
(Page 5)

Answer Key: Continued

- She will then need to be started on long-acting insulin like Lantus and short-acting insulin-like NovoLog for correction with meals.

Critical Thinking Check #6

- Unfortunately, at this time insulin is not available in pill form. It has to be taken via injection. Otherwise, it will not work correctly.

Critical Thinking Check #7

- Insulin vial with needles
- Insulin pen
- Insulin pump

Critical Thinking Check #8

- Miss Matthews should be taught how to count carbohydrates to determine the amount of insulin required.
- She should be given a prescribed sliding scale or insulin protocol to follow.
- She should be instructed on when to take her long-acting insulin and when to take regular insulin in relation to meal times. It is important that she does not take short-acting insulins without being ready to eat.
- Miss Matthews should be educated on the possibility of morning hyperglycemia due to the Somogyi effect or Dawn phenomenon, and be given suggestions to try an evening dose of insulin or an evening snack.
- The importance of follow-up appointments with her primary care provider and/or endocrinologist should be stressed. She should have her Hgb A1c checked every 3 months to start with.
- She should be educated on foods to avoid, such as desserts and sweets, beneficial foods, such as fruits and vegetables and high-quality proteins.
- She should carry candy or glucose tabs in case of a hypoglycemic reaction.

CUSHING'S DISEASE

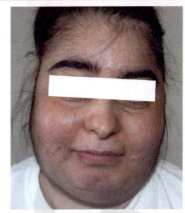

ByOzlem Celik, Mutlu Niyazoglu, Hikmet Soylu and Pinar Kadioglu - http://mrmjournal.biomedcentral.com/articles/10.1186/2049-6958-7-26, CC BY 2.5, https://commons.wikimedia.org/w/index.php?curid=47877333

Nursing Case Study #9
(Cushing's Disease)

Pathophysiology:
Similar to Cushing's syndrome which is much more common, Cushing's disease is a condition where the pituitary gland secretes too much hormone (ACTH) causing an overproduction of cortisol (stress hormone). It causes weight gain around the trunk and waist with fat loss in the less and arms. Patients may also develop a hump on the upper back that is caused by abnormal fat deposits. This disease weakens the immune system and can cause mood disorders such as anxiety and depression.

Patient:
Ms. Smith Is a 33 year old female who presents to her primary care provider for General muscle weakness and low back pain. She reports that this pain has been going on for about 3 months and the weakness has been getting worse over the last 2 weeks and she has been more fatigued with basic physical exertion. She reports getting "steroid injections" in her back previously, but they "didn't last long at all".

***Test your knowledge by referencing the answer key at the end of this study!

Critical Thinking Check #1   (Bloom's Taxonomy: Application)
What further history questions should be asked of Ms. Smith?

Ms. Smith has a history of Type II Diabetes and Asthma, and has been taking inhaled corticosteroids for the past 6 years. She also reports having irregular menstrual cycles for the past 2 years accompanied by unexplained weight gain in her abdomen. Her previous provider told her she might have Polycystic Ovarian Syndrome.

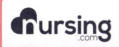

NURSING.com - "Tools and Confidence to Succeed in Nursing School."
©2023 TazKai LLC | NURSING.com - Reproduction Strictly Prohibited
Disclaimer information at NURSING.com

CUSHING'S DISEASE

Nursing Case Study #9
(Page 2)

Critical Thinking Check #2 *(Bloom's Taxonomy: Application)*
What initial nursing assessments should be performed?

Ms. Smith's Vital Signs were as follows:

- **HR** 78
- **BP** 156/92
- **RR** 14
- **Temp** 98.8°F

The nurse notes purple/pink stretch marks on arms, abdomen, and thighs. Ms. Smith has multiple cuts and bruises on her arms. When asked how she got them, she says "my skin is just so thin these days". She is obese with noticeable fatty deposits in the midsection and upper back.

Critical Thinking Check #3 *(Bloom's Taxonomy: Analysis)*
What diagnostic testing do you anticipate for Ms. Smith?

Ms. Smith is sent home with a pain reliever for her back pain while the laboratory results are processed. An ultrasound of her kidneys and ovaries is ordered, pending scheduling an appointment for next week. Two days later, lab values result and show the following:

- **Cortisol** 28 mg/dL (H)
- **Glucose** 265 mg/dL
- **K** 3.3 mEq/L
- **Na** 148 mg/dL
- **Ca** 7.8 mg/dL
- **Testosterone** levels elevated

CUSHING'S DISEASE

Nursing Case Study #9
(Page 3)

Critical Thinking Check #4   *(Bloom's Taxonomy: Analysis)*

Which finding(s) is/are concerning and need to be reported to the provider? Why?

Critical Thinking Check #5   *(Bloom's Taxonomy: Analysis)*

What do you believe is going on physiologically with Ms. Smith?

The provider notifies Ms. Smith that she needs to be seen again ASAP for further diagnostic testing to rule out any cardiac abnormalities. He tells her to stop taking her inhaled corticosteroid and prescribes a different rescue inhaler for her asthma. He also tells her she needs to begin taking some supplements, including calcium and potassium.

Critical Thinking Check #6   *(Bloom's Taxonomy: Analysis)*

Why does Ms. Smith need to have her heart checked out? What test would they do?

Critical Thinking Check #7   *(Bloom's Taxonomy: Analysis)*

Why does Ms. Smith need calcium supplements? What caused her hypocalcemia? How might this contribute to her back pain?

Critical Thinking Check #8   *(Bloom's Taxonomy: Analysis)*

Why does Ms. Smith have to stop taking her inhaler?

CUSHING'S DISEASE

 **Nursing Case Study #9
(Page 4)**

Answer Key:

💡 Critical Thinking Check #1:

- What medical history does she have?
- What medications does she take on a regular basis?
- What has she tried in the past for her back pain? What has worked?
- Is the pain associated with any specific activity or time of day? What makes it worse or makes it better?

💡 Critical Thinking Check #2:

- Heart and lung sounds
- Assess skin condition
- Assess strength x 4 extremities
- Abdominal assessment

💡 Critical Thinking Check #3:

- Complete Metabolic Panel – test electrolytes and kidney/liver function
- Hormone levels – estrogen, progesterone, testosterone, cortisol
- Complete Blood Count to evaluate immune system
- ESR and/or CRP to assess for inflammation

💡 Critical Thinking Check #4:

- Hypokalemia and hypernatremia can be detrimental to the cardiovascular and neurological system and need to be addressed quickly
- The elevated blood sugar and elevated cortisol levels combined with the clinical findings suggest possible Cushing's Syndrome

CUSHING'S DISEASE

Nursing Case Study #9
(Page 5)

Answer Key: Continued

💡 Critical Thinking Check #5

- Ms. Smith likely has developed Cushing's Syndrome due to chronic use of corticosteroids.
- This causes the Adrenal Glands to over-respond, secreting excess gluco-corticoids (hence the hyperglycemia and fat distribution), excess mineralo-corticoids (hence the electrolyte abnormalities), and excess androgens (hence the elevated testosterone levels).
- The hypocalcemia can also cause osteoporosis or soft, fragile bones

💡 Critical Thinking Check #6

- The hypokalemia can cause electrical abnormalities or arrhythmias
- She needs an EKG

💡 Critical Thinking Check #7

- Cushing's Syndrome causes hypocalcemia
- Hypocalcemia can cause calcium to be pulled from the bones to compensate – this creates an osteoporotic situation
- This may be why her back hurts – it is taking the weight of her body onto the soft, porous bones

💡 Critical Thinking Check #8

- The chronic use of the inhaled corticosteroids is the likely culprit – she should refer to her PCP or pulmonologist for other options to manage her asthma

BURN INJURY

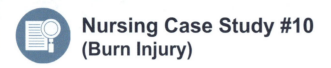

Nursing Case Study #10
(Burn Injury)

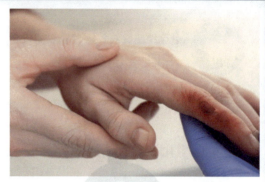

Pathophysiology:
A burn injury is tissue damage caused by heat, chemicals, electricity, radiation or sunlight. The degree of burn depends upon the depth and area that they cover. Deep burns heal slowly, can be difficult to treat and have a high risk of complications such as infection, amputation, and even death.

Patient:
Mr. Travis is a 32 year old male who presents to the ED after sustaining severe 2nd and 3rd degree burns in a house fire. The below diagram estimates his wounds. He weighs 85 kg and is 5'11".

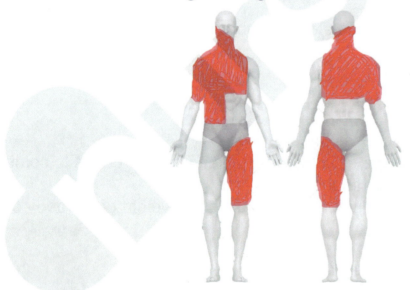

***Test your knowledge by referencing the answer key at the end of this study!

Critical Thinking Check #1 *(Bloom's Taxonomy: Application)*
Using the Rule of Nines, estimate the Total Body Surface Area Burned (TBSA %).

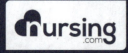

NURSING.com - "Tools and Confidence to Succeed in Nursing School."
©2023 TazKai LLC | NURSING.com - Reproduction Strictly Prohibited
Disclaimer information at NURSING.com

BURN INJURY

Nursing Case Study #10
(Page 2)

Critical Thinking Check #2 (Bloom's Taxonomy: Application)
Calculate the total fluid volume required for resuscitation in the first 24 hours using the Parkland Burn Formula.

Critical Thinking Check #3 (Bloom's Taxonomy: Analysis)
What is the TOP nursing priority for Mr. Travis?

You note circumferential burns around the Right Upper Arm and soot around the mouth with singed nose hairs, plus some facial swelling.

Critical Thinking Check #4 (Bloom's Taxonomy: Analysis)
What are your main concerns for complication(s)?

Critical Thinking Check #5 (Bloom's Taxonomy: Analysis)
Physiologically, explain the alterations in Mr. Travis's vital signs.

Critical Thinking Check #6 (Bloom's Taxonomy: Analysis)
How will you know if fluid resuscitation is effective?

Mr. Travis is intubated for airway protection and taken to the OR for surgical debridement of his burns. He is then transferred to the Burn ICU

BURN INJURY

 Nursing Case Study #10
(Page 3)

Critical Thinking Check #7 *(Bloom's Taxonomy: Analysis)*

What are priorities for daily care of Mr. Travis?

Critical Thinking Check #8 *(Bloom's Taxonomy: Comprehension)*

Mr. Travis will need skin grafts. How will you explain autologous skin grafts to Mr. Travis and his family?

Answer Key:

Critical Thinking Check #1:

- Half of the head/neck – 4.5%
- Top half of front torso – 9%
- Top half of back – 9%
- Full top half of right arm – 4.5%
- Full top half of left leg – 9%
- Half of front abdomen – 4.5%
- Half of lower back – 4.5%
- TOTAL – 45%

Critical Thinking Check #2:

- 4 x 45% x 85 kg = 15,300 mL in 24 hours
- Give ½ in the first 8 hours = Start fluids at 956 mL/hr

Critical Thinking Check #3:

- Fluid resuscitation to prevent hypovolemic shock
- Mr. Travis's vitals are: BP 90/48, HR 108, Temp 97.2, Pain 10/10.

BURN INJURY

 Nursing Case Study #10
(Page 4)

Answer Key:

Critical Thinking Check #4:

- Airway due to possible/likely inhalation burns and airway swelling
- Compartment syndrome due to circumferential burns around right arm

Critical Thinking Check #5:

- He is likely hypovolemic due to the loss of fluids from the burns, hence the low BP and high HR
- He is hypothermic because of his inability to regulate temperature due to
- skin loss

Critical Thinking Check #6:

- Fluid resuscitation should be titrated to urine output of at least 0.5 mL/kg/hr or 30-50 mL/hr
- If excess urine output, slow fluids
- If not enough, speed up fluids

Critical Thinking Check #7:

- Infection prevention and meticulous wound care – sterile dressing changes
- Pain control – PCA if able
- Manage ventilator and respiratory needs until able to be extubated
- Maintain temperature and hemodynamics

Critical Thinking Check #8:

- Autologous skin grafts are performed by taking a slice of healthy tissue from somewhere else on the patient's body, for example, his right thigh that isn't burned, and then running it through a meshing device.

BURN INJURY

Nursing Case Study #10
(Page 5)

Answer Key: Continued

- This allows it to be stretched over the wound and secured in place, then the skin will grow in around the graft

BREAST CANCER

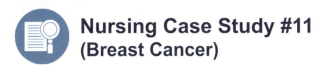

Nursing Case Study #11 (Breast Cancer)

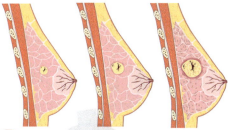

Breast cancer

Laboratoires Servier, CC BY-SA 3.0 <https://creativecommons.org/licenses/by-sa/3.0>, via Wikimedia Commons

Pathophysiology:
Breast cancer is cancer that develops from breast tissue. Signs of breast cancer may include a lump in the breast, a change in breast shape, skin dimpling, milk rejection, fluid from the nipple, a newly inverted nipple, or a red or scaly patch of skin. In those with distant spread of the disease, there may be bone pain, swollen lymph nodes, shortness of breath, or yellow skin.

Breast cancer is the second most common cancer diagnosed in women in the United States. Breast cancer can occur in both men and women, but it's far more common in women.

Patient:
Natasha is a 32-year-old female African American patient arriving at the surgery oncology unit status post left breast mastectomy and lymph node excision. She arrives from the post-anesthesia unit (PACU) via hospital bed with her spouse, Angelica, at the bedside. They explain that a self-exam revealed a lump, and, after mammography and biopsy, this surgery was the next step in cancer treatment, and they have an oncologist they trust. Natasha says, "I wonder how I will look later since I want reconstruction."

***Test your knowledge by referencing the answer key at the end of this study!

Critical Thinking Check #1	*(Bloom's Taxonomy: Apply)*
What assessments and initial check-in activities should the nurse perform for this post-operative patient?	

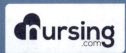

BREAST CANCER

Nursing Case Study #11
(Page 2)

Critical Thinking Check #2   *(Bloom's Taxonomy: Analyze)*
What orders does the nurse expect to see in the chart?

After screening and assessing the patient, the nurse finds she is AAOx4 (awake, alert and oriented to date, place, person and situation). The PACU staff gave her ice due to dry mouth which she self-administers and tolerates well. She has a 20G IV in her right hand. She states her pain is 2 on a scale of 1-10 with 10 being the highest. Her wife asks when the patient can eat and about visiting hours. Natasha also asks about a bedside commode for urination and why she does not have a "pain medicine button". Another call light goes off and the nurse's clinical communicator (unit issued cell phone) rings.

The nurse heard in a report about a Jackson-Pratt drain but there are no dressing change instructions, so she does not further assess the post-op dressing situation in order to deal with everything going on at the moment. She then sits down to document this patient.

Medications ordered in electronic health record but not yet administered by PACU:
- Tramadol 50 mg q 6 hrs. Prn for mild to moderate pain.
- Oxycodone 5 mg PO q 4 hrs. Prn for moderate to severe pain (5-7 on 1-10 scale)
- Fentanyl 25 mcg IV q3hrs. Prn For breakthrough pain (no relieve from PO meds or greater than 8 on 1-10 scale)
- Lactated Ringers 125 mL/hr IV infusion, continuous x 2 liters
- Naloxone 0.4-2 mg IV/IM/SC; may repeat q2-3min PRN respiratory rate less than 6 bpm; not to exceed 10 mg

- **BP** 110/70 SpO2 98% on Room Air
- **HR** 68 bpm and regular Ht 157 cm

BREAST CANCER

Nursing Case Study #11
(Page 3)

- **RR** 14 bpm Wt 53 kg
- **Temp** 36.°5C EBL 130mL
- **CBC** -WNL
- **BMP- K** 5.4
- **Potassium** – 5.4 mEq/L

Critical Thinking Check #3	(Bloom's Taxonomy: Apply)
What education should be conducted regarding post-op medications?	

Critical Thinking Check #4	(Bloom's Taxonomy: Evaluate)
What are some medical and/or non-medical concerns the nurse may have at this point? If there are any, should they be brought up to the surgeon?	

Natasha sleeps through the night with no complaints of pain. Lab comes to draw the ordered labs and the CNA takes vital signs. See below:

CBC
- **HGB** 7.2 g/dl
- **HCT** 21.6%

BMP
- **Sodium** 130 mEq/L
- **Potassium** 6.0 mEq/L
- **BUN** 5 mg/dL
- **BP** 84/46
- **SpO2** 91% on Room Air
- **HR** 109 RR 22 bpm

BREAST CANCER

Nursing Case Study #11
(Page 4)

Critical Thinking Check #5   *(Bloom's Taxonomy: Analyze)*

What should the nurse do FIRST? Is the nurse concerned about the AM labs? AM vital signs? Why or why not?

Check the dressing and drain for BLEEDING (assess the patient). The patient should also sit up and allow staff to check the bed for signs of bleeding. Reinforce the dressing as needed. Record output from the drain (or review documentation of all the night's drain output). Labs and vital signs indicate she may be losing blood.

Critical Thinking Check #6   *(Bloom's Taxonomy: Apply)*

What orders does the nurse anticipate from the surgeon?

Critical Thinking Check #7   *(Bloom's Taxonomy: Analyze)*

How should the nurse address Natasha's declaration? What alerts the nurse to a possible complication?

The surgeon orders 1 unit packed red blood cells to be infused. The nurse then goes to the patient to ask about religious affiliation and to discuss the doctor's order. After verifying that Natasha is not a practicing Jehovah's Witness, the nurse proceeds to prepare the transfusion.

Critical Thinking Check #8   *(Bloom's Taxonomy: Apply)*

What is required to administer blood or blood products?

BREAST CANCER

Nursing Case Study #11
(Page 5)

After receiving one unit of packed red blood cells (PRBC), Natasha rests quietly but still appears upset. The nurse asks if she needs anything and Natasha states, "Yes. What happens when I get out of here? I am so worried about what is next."

Critical Thinking Check #9	(Bloom's Taxonomy: Apply)
How should the nurse respond to this question?	

Answer Key:

 Critical Thinking Check #1:

- Airway patency, respiratory rate (RR), peripheral oxygen saturation (SpO2), heart rate (HR), blood pressure (BP), mental status, temperature, and the presence of pain, nausea, or vomiting are assessed upon arrival. Medication allergies, social questioning (i.e. living situation, religious affiliation), as well as education preference are also vital. An admission assessment MUST include an examination of the post-op dressing and any drains in place. This should be documented accordingly.
- The hand-off should be thorough and may be standardized. Some institutions have implemented a formal checklist to provide a structure for the intra-hospital transfer of surgical patients. Such instruments help to standardize processes thereby ensuring that clinicians have critical information when patient care is transferred to a new team. The nurse should also prepare to provide education based on surgeon AND oncologist guidance.

Critical Thinking Check #2:

- Post-op medications, dressing change and/or drain management, strict I&O, no BP/stick on the operative side (rationale is to help prevent lymphedema – Blood pressure (BP) measurement with a cuff on the ipsilateral arm has

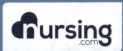

BREAST CANCER

Nursing Case Study #11
(Page 6)

Answer Key: Continued

- been posed as a risk factor for the development of LE after-breast cancer therapy for years, regardless of the amount of lymph node excision.)
- Parameters for calling the surgeon are also important. The nurse should also check for an oncology service consult.

Critical Thinking Check #3:

- New post-op pain guidelines rely less on patient-controlled analgesia (aka "pain medicine button") than in previous years. Most facilities will have an approved standing protocol (i.e., "Multimodal analgesia and Opioid Prescribing recommendation" guideline) or standing orders. The patient must be instructed on how to rate pain using facility-approved tools (aka "pain scales"). She should also report any medication-related side effects and reinforce there is a reversal medication in case of an opioid overdose.

Critical Thinking Check #4:

- The nurse may request an anti-emetic such as ondansetron 4 mg IV q 6 hrs prn nausea vomiting (N&V) since it is not uncommon post-op for the patient to have N&V. The rate of LR is a little high for such a small patient and could cause electrolyte imbalances.
- The nurse may also inquire about the oncologist being on the case and ask if the surgeon has discussed reconstruction with the patient yet. She may also want to ask about dressing change orders.

Critical Thinking Check #5:

- Check the dressing and drain for bleeding (assess the patient). The patient should also sit up and allow staff to check the bed for signs of bleeding. Reinforce the dressing as needed. Record output from the drain (or review documentation of the night's drain output). Labs and vital signs indicate

BREAST CANCER

Nursing Case Study #11
(Page 7)

Answer Key: Continued

- she may be losing blood.

💡 Critical Thinking Check #6:

- The nurse should expect an order to transfuse blood for this patient. Also, dressing reinforcement or change instructions are needed in the case of saturation)

💡 Critical Thinking Check #7:

- First, the complication is that "Kingdom Hall" is the site of worship for Jehovah's Witnesses. They do not accept ANY blood product, not even in emergencies. It is vital the nurse determines the patient's affiliation and religious exceptions for medical care before moving forward. Next, employ therapeutic communication to elicit more details about Natasha's concerns. Say things like, "tell me why you think you're not attractive?" She may discuss reconstruction options or ask the patient to write down specific questions about this option to ask the provider later. Ask about getting family in to provide support. Seek information to give the patient about support groups and other resources available (as appropriate, ie. prosthetics, special undergarments/accessories, etc)

💡 Critical Thinking Check #8:

- First, the patient's CONSENT is required to give blood products. The nurse must also prepare to stay with the patient for at least the first 15 minutes of the transfusion taking a baseline set of V/S prior to infusion. Then, V/S per protocol (frequent). Education is also required. The patient should report feeling flushed, back or flank pain, shortness of breath, chest pain, chills, itching, hives. Normal saline ONLY for infusion setup and flushing: size IV 20g or higher. Always defer infusion time limits to "per policy" because this

BREAST CANCER

Nursing Case Study #11
(Page 8)

Answer Key: Continued

- can differ vastly

💡 Critical Thinking Check #9:

- Planning for post-op cancer treatment should have begun prior to the surgery. Ask the patient if she has discussed plans with her oncologist. Refer to any specialist documentation to see if this is mentioned. Remind the patient of the specialist's assessment and planning information. Reinforce that testing of the tissue may change the course of treatment as well. Provide education AS PER THE PATIENT'S STATED PREFERENCE and/or resources based on what the plan includes (ie. chemotherapy, radiation, further surgery. Continually assess and reassess patient understanding. Include family and/or support with the patient's approval.

HYPERTHYROIDISM

Nursing Case Study #12
(Hyperthyroidism)

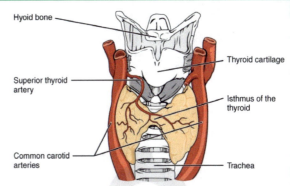

Pathophysiology:

Hyperthyroidism is a condition of excess secretion of thyroid hormones, we'll see increased levels of T3, T4, and Free T4 in the blood. We'll also see decreased levels of TSH, or Thyroid Stimulating Hormone. Why is that? Well, let's review how these hormones get secreted. The hypothalamus in the brain releases Thyrotropin Releasing Hormone, which goes to the pituitary gland and tells it to release Thyroid Stimulating Hormone. TSH goes to the Thyroid gland to tell it to secrete more thyroid hormones. Then, when the levels are high enough, the body sends a signal back to the hypothalamus to tell it to stop. That's called a negative feedback loop.

Patient:

Mrs. Black is a 31 year old female who is 2 weeks postpartum. This morning her husband found her difficult to rouse and confused, and called 911. The husband indicates she has been quite anxious since the birth of their first child. He reports she has had nausea and vomiting for two days, as well as watery diarrhea and generalized abdominal pain. She hasn't been able to breastfeed baby because she's been too anxious. Husband denies any sick contacts or recent travel.

***Test your knowledge by referencing the answer key at the end of this study!**

Critical Thinking Check #1   (Bloom's Taxonomy: Apply)
What other medical history would you want to attempt to gather from the husband?

HYPERTHYROIDISM

Nursing Case Study #12
(Page 2)

Critical Thinking Check #2   *(Bloom's Taxonomy: Apply)*

What initial nursing assessments should be performed?

Upon further questioning, the husband reports Mrs. Black has a history of Hyperlipidemia, Graves Disease, and asthma and takes simvastatin and propylthiouracil daily, plus her rescue inhaler when she needs it. Upon assessment, Mrs. Black is somnolent and only minimally responsive to painful stimuli. She is unable to answer orientation questions and just keeps repeating her husband's name. The nurse notes redness to her eyes and swelling around her eyelids. Heart rate is rapid and irregular. Lungs have diffuse crackles bilaterally. Vital signs are as follows:

- **HR** 145 bpm
- **BP** 120/76 mmHg
- **RR** 32 bpm
- **Temp** 101°F
- **SpO2** 89% on 4L nasal cannula

Critical Thinking Check #3   *(Bloom's Taxonomy: Analyze)*

What should the nurse's first action be?

Critical Thinking Check #4   *(Bloom's Taxonomy: Analyze)*

Based on the information you have, what diagnostic laboratory tests would you anticipate the provider ordering?

HYPERTHYROIDISM

Nursing Case Study #12
(Page 3)

- **RR** 14 bpm Wt 53 kg
- **Temp** 36.°5C EBL 130mL
- **CBC** -WNL
- **BMP- K** 5.4
- **Potassium** – 5.4 mEq/L

Critical Thinking Check #3	(Bloom's Taxonomy: Apply)

What education should be conducted regarding post-op medications?

Critical Thinking Check #4	(Bloom's Taxonomy: Evaluate)

What are some medical and/or non-medical concerns the nurse may have at this point? If there are any, should they be brought up to the surgeon?

Mrs. Black becomes more obtunded and her heart rate goes up to 155. The provider orders a 12-lead EKG and proceeds to prepare for intubation for airway protection. The Respiratory Therapist comes to the bedside and notes the patient has a swollen thyroid gland. For this reason, the Anesthesia team is called to the bedside to assist in a successful intubation. The provider orders a full lab panel, including CBC, CMP, LFTs, and a Thyroid Panel, plus an Arterial Blood Gas, and consults the ICU team to admit Mrs. Black.

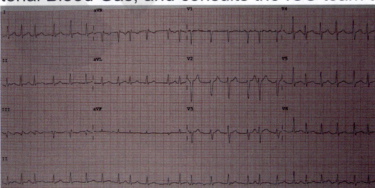

James Heilman, MD, CC BY-SA 3.0 <https://creativecommons.org/licenses/by-sa/3.0>, via Wikimedia Commons

HYPERTHYROIDISM

Nursing Case Study #12
(Page 4)

Critical Thinking Check #5   (Bloom's Taxonomy: Analyze)

Interpret this EKG. What are the implications of this rhythm for the patient?

Critical Thinking Check #6   (Bloom's Taxonomy: Analyze)

What could this mean?

Lab results return on Mrs. Black as she is transferred to the ICU:

- **Na** 144
- **pH** 7.33
- **TSH** 0.1
- **K** 5.0
- **pCO2** 48
- **WBC** 14K
- **Mg** 1.0
- **HCO3–** 24
- **Hgb** 12.5
- **BUN** 11
- **pO2** 190
- **Hct** 38%
- **Cr** 0.7
- **Lactate** 3.2
- **Plt** 450K

Critical Thinking Check #7   (Bloom's Taxonomy: Analyze)

What is going on physiologically with Mrs. Black?

HYPERTHYROIDISM

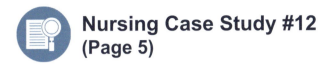

Nursing Case Study #12
(Page 5)

Critical Thinking Check #8 *(Bloom's Taxonomy: Analyze)*

What medications do you anticipate the provider ordering for Mrs. Black?

The provider orders a beta blocker and IV fluids for Mrs. Black, as well as an increased dose of propylthiouracil (PTU). She is stable for now, but it may take a few days for her to overcome this thyroid storm/crisis. Her husband asks the nurse what caused this.

Critical Thinking Check #9 *(Bloom's Taxonomy: Analyze)*

What is the best response to the husband to explain what triggered Mrs. Black's Thyroid Storm/Crisis?

Answer Key:

 Critical Thinking Check #1:

- Any complications with the pregnancy or delivery?
- Characteristics of vomit/diarrhea? Any bleeding?
- Medical conditions
- Medications taken on a daily basis
- Allergies

 Critical Thinking Check #2:

- Neuro assessment – Level of consciousness, pupils, strength/movements
- Abdominal assessment due to diarrhea and vomiting, assess for any masses, tenderness, or guarding with palpation
- Full set of vital signs
- Skin assessment – color, temperature, condition

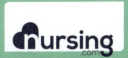

HYPERTHYROIDISM

Nursing Case Study #12
(Page 6)

Answer Key: Continued

- Heat and lung sounds and respiratory/airway status.

💡 Critical Thinking Check #3:

- Neuro assessment – Level of consciousness, pupils, strength/movements
- Abdominal assessment due to diarrhea and vomiting, assess for any masses, tenderness, or guarding with palpation
- Full set of vital signs
- Skin assessment – color, temperature, condition
- Heat and lung sounds and respiratory/airway status

💡 Critical Thinking Check #4:

- Full metabolic panel for electrolytes, renal function, etc.
- Thyroid panel
- Complete blood count to assess for infection or occult bleeding
- Arterial Blood Gas to assess oxygenation / ventilation / gas exchange

💡 Critical Thinking Check #5:

- Atrial Fibrillation with Rapid Ventricular Response (rapid rate, >150)
- This severe tachycardia with arrhythmia can be detrimental to the patient's cardiac output, especially if this is not her baseline
- It may also indicate underlying electrolyte abnormalities and/or other hormonal changes that are causing the severe tachycardia
- No one's heart can tolerate this fast blood pressure for that long

💡 Critical Thinking Check #6:

- Mrs. Black likely has a large goiter, this could cause obstruction of the airway and create for a difficult intubation.

HYPERTHYROIDISM

Nursing Case Study #12
(Page 7)

Answer Key: Continued

- The Anesthesia team is considered the expert consultants for airways within the hospital, most times. They are not only experts, but they can also bring equipment with them to assist with more difficult airways

Critical Thinking Check #7:

- Mrs. Black is likely experiencing a Thyroid Storm or Thyroid Crisis. This causes severe tachycardia and arrhythmias, N/V/D, and a severe febrile state.
- Remember hyperthyroidism is 'hypermetabolic' – so now those things have become severe
- The low TSH level is the clue that her thyroid hormone levels are likely sky high, you can count on that, even without the actual Thyroxine levels.

Critical Thinking Check #8:

- Beta blocker or calcium channel blocker to address the hypertension and tachycardia
- Propylthiouracil or methimazole as antithyroid therapy
- Any other medications required to address the symptoms during the crisis (antipyretics, antidiarrheals, antiemetics, etc.)

Critical Thinking Check #9:

- The stress of the pregnancy and delivery are likely the initial trigger.
- The start of the Thyroid Crisis will have caused some anxiety for her and then continued to be further exacerbated due to excess stress

BIPOLAR DISORDER

Nursing Case Study #13
(Bipolar Disorder)

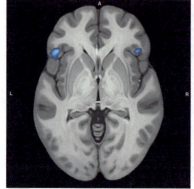
Petergstrom, CC BY-SA 4.0 <https://creativecommons.org/licenses/by-sa/4.0>, via Wikimedia Commons

Pathophysiology:
Bipolar disorder is classified as a mood disorder. Mood disorders are a category of mental illnesses that affect a person's emotional state over a long period of time. Emotions, or moods may fluctuate frequently and seemingly without any reason. Clients with mood disorders are at a higher risk for substance abuse and suicidal tendencies. Treatment is geared toward managing symptoms through the use of medications and psychotherapy.

Patient:
Kelli is a 20-year-old patient brought to the ER after being reported by neighbors in her apartment complex for disruptive behavior. Law enforcement and emergency medical services were called, and, as a team, decided she needed a higher level of medical care.

The patient says she is" on a break from art college" but works at a local restaurant as a server and occasionally cleans houses as well. She has also sold her paintings and drawings in the past as well. She denies taking any medication. She also says, "I don't understand why I am here. I was working on my art projects, and I guess I played my music too loud or something. I said I'd come here so I would not be arrested."

***Test your knowledge by referencing the answer key at the end of this study!

Critical Thinking Check #1   *(Bloom's Taxonomy: Apply)*
What are some questions that should be included in the initial assessment?

BIPOLAR DISORDER

Nursing Case Study #13
(Page 2)

Critical Thinking Check #2   *(Bloom's Taxonomy: Analyze)*

What interventions do you anticipate being ordered by the provider?

Kelli's drug and alcohol tests are negative. Her roommate is now at the bedside and asks to speak to staff privately. She expresses concern that Kelli can be emotional at times as well as going days without sleep then not being able to get out of bed. The nurse returns to further evaluate the patient.

Critical Thinking Check #3   *(Bloom's Taxonomy: Apply)*

With this new information, what might the nurse ask Kelli?

Kelli admits to being able to stay awake for what seems like entire weekends without being tired, but that is when she says her creativity is best. When she was attending college and living in the dorms, she says she had lots of friends but worried about what she calls "all the partying." This is because she liked to "hook up" with strangers because it was fun, but she worries about possible sexually transmitted infections now that she is older. She says she was extremely popular, and her talent was at its peak. But there are times she could not pay attention in class or even get out of bed, so she dropped out of school. Sometimes, she cannot even touch her art supplies, but says she is probably the "most talented artist around."

Critical Thinking Check #4   *(Bloom's Taxonomy: Apply)*

What signs and symptoms indicate Kelli may have bipolar disorder?

BIPOLAR DISORDER

Nursing Case Study #13
(Page 3)

Critical Thinking Check #5   (Bloom's Taxonomy: Understand)
Are there risk factors for this condition?

Kelli's medical records have arrived, and the provider advises nursing staff she has a history of being brought to the ER for similar episodes. The provider says, "This patient is a schizophrenic. We don't have time for this."

Critical Thinking Check #6   (Bloom's Taxonomy: Evaluate)
What is the best response to the provider's statement?

Kelli rests quietly in the exam room with her roommate at the bedside. She asks, "Can someone help me get better? I am tired of this. I am such a burden on everyone."

Critical Thinking Check #7   (Bloom's Taxonomy: Evaluate)
What should the nurse screen Kelli for at this point?

Critical Thinking Check #8   (Bloom's Taxonomy: Apply)
How can the nurse address Kelli's question about help?

Kelli is amenable to being held for the state's required psychological hold. She says she wants to be able to live her life as "normally" as possible. She asks about medications that may be available to help.

BIPOLAR DISORDER

Nursing Case Study #13
(Page 4)

Critical Thinking Check #9   (Bloom's Taxonomy: Apply)
What patient education about medications should the nurse provide at this time?

Critical Thinking Check #10   (Bloom's Taxonomy: Understand)
The nurse knows which medications may be prescribed for long-term management of this condition?

Answer Key:

Critical Thinking Check #1:

- Ask about drug and alcohol consumption and previous episodes. Make sure she does not intend to harm herself or others. Check to see why the patient does not understand coming to a medical treatment facility (make sure she is lucid). Ask about trauma or accidents.

Critical Thinking Check #2:

- Obtain old medical charts (there may be a pattern). Screen for drugs and alcohol. Assess for trauma (especially head injury, so neuro checks). Complete a thorough medical history to rule out medical reasons for behavior. Conduct a medical examination including labs (eg. thyroid-stimulating hormone, complete blood count, chemistries)

Critical Thinking Check #3:

- Ask about "periods of unusually intense emotion, changes in sleep patterns and activity levels, and uncharacteristic behavior—often without recognizing

BIPOLAR DISORDER

Nursing Case Study #13
(Page 5)

Answer Key: Continued

- their likely harmful or undesirable effects" (from NIH). Dig deeper to find if these "episodes" last for long or short periods. Specifically, ask about extreme highs and lows, change in appetite, racing thoughts vs concentration difficulty, risky behaviors (eg gambling, extreme shopping sprees, sexual promiscuity), anxiety, excessive talking, thoughts of death/dying.

Critical Thinking Check #4:

- Sleep disturbances, cycling between being creative and not being able to concentrate, sexual promiscuity, feelings of grandiosity, loss of pleasure of usual activities

Critical Thinking Check #5:

- The exact cause of bipolar disorder is not clear. The problem may be related to an imbalance of chemicals in the brain such as norepinephrine, serotonin, or dopamine. These chemicals allow cells to communicate with each other and play an essential role in all brain functions, including movement, sensation, memory, and emotions.
- Approximately one to three percent of people worldwide have bipolar disorder. People with a family history of bipolar disorder are at increased risk of developing the condition. Most people develop the first symptoms of bipolar disorder between age 15 to 30 years.

Critical Thinking Check #6:

- As the patient's advocate, the nurse should advise the provider this is inappropriate. First, it is a disparaging remark. Second, if he means schizophrenic, that is not accurate and as an ER physician should refer the patient for further psychiatric screening and evaluation.

BIPOLAR DISORDER

Nursing Case Study #13
(Page 6)

Answer Key: Continued

- It is never wrong to stand up to providers or colleagues, but it should be done respectfully and NOT in front of the patient when at all possible.

💡 Critical Thinking Check #7:

- Suicidal ideations include whether she has a plan or has attempted suicide in the past. Suicide screening is an ongoing process and not just a few questions at admission. Per UpToDate, "A review estimated that approximately 10 to 15 percent of bipolar patients die by suicide and many studies indicate that the rate of suicide deaths in patients is greater than the rate in the general population."

💡 Critical Thinking Check #8:

- Something like (from uptodate), "Treatment of mania focuses on managing symptoms and keeping you safe. In the early phase of mania (called the acute phase), you may be psychotic (having false, fixed beliefs or hearing voices or seeing things others cannot see or hear). You may not be able to make good decisions and you may be at risk of hurting yourself or others. You may need to be treated in a hospital temporarily, until your medicine begins to work."
- Also, "Once the worst symptoms of mania or depression are under control, treatment focuses on preventing a recurrence. People who have suffered a manic episode are often advised to continue taking medicine(s) to control bipolar disorder. Although medicines are the treatment of choice for bipolar disorder, counseling and talk therapy also have an important role in treatment. This is especially true after an acute episode has passed. Psychotherapy may include individual counseling as well as education, marital and family therapy, or treatment of alcohol and/or drug abuse. Therapy can help you to stick with your medicine, which can decrease the risk of relapse and the need for hospitalization."

BIPOLAR DISORDER

 Nursing Case Study #13
(Page 7)

Answer Key: Continued

💡 **Critical Thinking Check #9:**

- While it is beyond the scope of the RN to prescribe medications, generalized education on pharmaceutical options is acceptable. Saying something like, "Treatments with medications is recommended for people with bipolar disorder, and studies show starting it early and maintaining it is best." Point out there may be multiple medications needed and they may need to be changed and/or adjusted for her individual responses.

💡 **Critical Thinking Check #10:**

- Mood stabilizers (examples: lithium, valproic acid, divalproex sodium,
- carbamazepine, and lamotrigine). Antipsychotics. [examples: olanzapine (Zyprexa), risperidone (Risperdal), quetiapine (Seroquel), aripiprazole (Abilify), ziprasidone (Geodon), lurasidone (Latuda) or asenapine (Saphris)]
- Antidepressants or antidepressant-antipsychotic combo like Symbyax combines the antidepressant fluoxetine and the antipsychotic olanzapine
- Anti-anxiety medications (example: benzodiazepines)

SEPTIC SHOCK

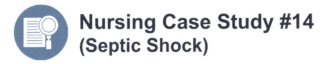

**Nursing Case Study #14
(Septic Shock)**

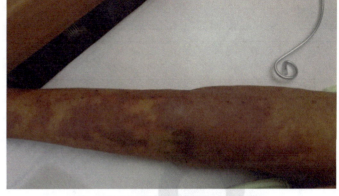

Emergency doc, CC BY-SA 4.0 <https://creativecommons.org/licenses/by-sa/4.0>, via Wikimedia Commons

Pathophysiology:
Septic shock is a severe medical condition that occurs when the body's response to infection goes haywire, leading to life-threatening complications. It starts with an infection, often caused by bacteria, entering the bloodstream. Normally, the immune system fights off the infection by releasing chemicals to combat the invading pathogens. However, in septic shock, the body's response becomes exaggerated and uncontrolled. These chemicals, including cytokines and other inflammatory molecules, flood the body, causing widespread inflammation. This excessive inflammation leads to a cascade of events, such as dilated blood vessels, reduced blood flow to vital organs, and impaired oxygen delivery to tissues. As a result, multiple organs, like the heart, lungs, kidneys, and liver, begin to malfunction, potentially causing organ failure. Early recognition and prompt medical intervention are crucial in managing septic shock to prevent further complications and improve patient outcomes.

Patient:
This septic shock case study is designed to help the nursing student better understand nursing care for a patient with sepsis. Mr. McMillan, a 92-year old male, presents to the Emergency Department (ED) with urinary hesitancy and burning and a fever at home of 101.6°F. His caregiver states "he just doesn't seem like himself".

***Test your knowledge by referencing the answer key at the end of this study!*

Critical Thinking Check #1   *(Bloom's Taxonomy: Apply)*
What initial nursing assessments need to be performed for Mr. McMillan?

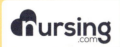

SEPTIC SHOCK

Nursing Case Study #14
(Page 2)

Critical Thinking Check #2 *(Bloom's Taxonomy: Analyze)*

What diagnostic tests should be ordered for Mr. McMillan?

Critical Thinking Check #3 *(Bloom's Taxonomy: Apply)*

What nursing actions would you take at this time for Mr. McMillan? Why?

The ED provider orders the following:

- Bloodwork – CBC, BMP, ABG, Lactic Acid, Blood Cultures x 2
- Urine Tests – Urinalysis, Urine Culture
- Diagnostics – CXR (chest x-ray), KUB (x-ray of kidneys, ureters, and bladder)
- Nasal Cannula to keep SpO2> 92%
- Meds – 1L Normal Saline bolus IV x 1, now. 1,500 mg Vancomycin IVPB x 1 dose, now

Critical Thinking Check #4 *(Bloom's Taxonomy: Analyze)*

Which order should you implement first? Why?

All blood and urine tests are completed and you initiate the fluid bolus for Mr. McMillan. You are still waiting for the Vancomycin to arrive from the pharmacy. You notice he is more drowsy. He is now only oriented to self and feels warmer. You take another set of vital signs to find the following:
- **BP** 86/50 mmHg MAP 62 mmHg
- **HR** 108 bpm Temp 39.3°C
- **RR** 36 bpm SpO2 88% on Room Air

SEPTIC SHOCK

Nursing Case Study #14
(Page 3)

Mr. McMillan's lab results have also resulted, the following abnormal values were reported:

- **WBC** 22,000 / mcL Lactic Acid 3.6 mmol/L
- **pH** 7.22 pCO2 30 mmHg
- **HCO3** 16 mEq/L pO2 64 mmHg

Critical Thinking Check #5	(Bloom's Taxonomy: Apply)
What action(s) should you take at this time? Why?	

Critical Thinking Check #6	(Bloom's Taxonomy: Analyze)
What orders do you anticipate for Mr. McMillan? (procedures, meds, transfer, etc?)	

Mr. McMillan responds well to the first liter of fluids, and antibiotics are initiated within an hour of arrival. The ED physicians place an arterial line and central line to initiate vasopressors. They order a Norepinephrine infusion to be titrated to keep MAP > 65 mmHg. The Critical Care team asks you to prepare the patient for transfer to the ICU.

- **Art. Line BP** 82/48 mmHg
- **MAP** 58 mmHg
- **HR** 122 bpm
- **CVP** 4 mmHg
- **RR** 32 bpm
- **SVR** 640 dynes/sec/m-5
- **SpO2** 90% on Room Air

SEPTIC SHOCK

Nursing Case Study #14
(Page 4)

Critical Thinking Check #7 *(Bloom's Taxonomy: Analyze)*
What, physiologically, is going on with Mr. McMillan?

Critical Thinking Check #8 *(Bloom's Taxonomy: Comprehend)*
What does it mean to titrate an infusion to keep MAP >65?

After 2 days in the ICU, a norepinephrine infusion and a total of two liters of normal saline, Mr. McMillan's blood pressure is stable, his MAP is 67 mmHg. He is becoming more alert and is now oriented to person, place, and time. His blood and urine cultures were positive for bacterial growth. He has received multiple doses of Vancomycin as well as antibiotics targeted to his specific bacterial infection. He is being weaned off of the vasopressors, and the providers hope he can transfer out of the ICU tomorrow.

Critical Thinking Check #9 *(Bloom's Taxonomy: Apply)*
What explanation or education topics would you want to provide to the patient and his caregiver before discharge?

Answer Key:

Critical Thinking Check #1:

- Full set vital signs (T, P, RR, BP, SpO2)
- OLDCARTS or PQRST assessment of symptoms (urinary burning)
- LOC/orientation assessment
- Heart and lung sounds

SEPTIC SHOCK

Nursing Case Study #14
(Page 5)

Answer Key: Continued

💡 Critical Thinking Check #2:

- Blood Tests – CBC, BMP, ABG, Lactic Acid, Blood Cultures x 2
- Urine Tests – Urinalysis, Urine Culture
- X-rays – Chest, Kidneys/Ureters/Bladder

💡 Critical Thinking Check #3:

- Elevate the HOB to improve breathing and oxygenation
- Apply cardiac monitor
- Notify provider of elevated temp and low SpO2
- Apply cool washcloth to forehead and/or behind neck for comfort
- Possibly get ice packs to axillae and groin and remove any blankets to help bring the patient's temperature closer to normal.

💡 Critical Thinking Check #4:

- Blood and urine cultures must be drawn before any antibiotics are administered.
- Blood work – urine tests – fluids – antibiotics
- IF the patient's SpO2 is below 92%, apply oxygen via nasal cannula – at this time, there is no indication of that, yet.

💡 Critical Thinking Check #5:

- #1 – apply oxygen via nasal cannula – ensure HOB elevated for easy breathing
- Notify provider of decreasing blood pressure and elevated WBC, lactic acid

SEPTIC SHOCK

Nursing Case Study #14
(Page 6)

Answer Key: Continued

Critical Thinking Check #6:

- Mr. McMillan may need another liter of IV fluids. The guidelines are for patients to receive 30 mL/kg of body weight in the first 6 hours. That means he would need to receive at least 1,800 mL of IV fluid bonuses.
- Mr. McMillan may need vasopressors to improve his blood pressure – in which case he will also need a central line for administration of those medications as well as an arterial line to monitor his MAP.
- Mr. McMillan will need to be transferred to the ICU for close monitoring and management of his drips

Critical Thinking Check #7:

- Mr. McMillan has an infection, likely urinary, and it has created a systemic inflammatory response. That inflammatory response is causing massive peripheral vasodilation so his vital organs are not receiving adequate blood flow
- He is showing signs of decreased perfusion to his brain (↓ LOC) and decreased cardiac output (↓ BP).
- His skin is warm and flushed and his temperature is elevated because of the vasodilation in the non-vital organs.

Critical Thinking Check #8:

- Titration means achieving the desired result with the least amount of drug possible. Therefore we would adjust the infusion up or down to maintain the MAP above, but not too far above, 65 mmHg

SEPTIC SHOCK

Nursing Case Study #14
(Page 7)

Answer Key: Continued

Critical Thinking Check #9:

- Sepsis and septic shock are a result of a severe infection that has gotten into the bloodstream and affected the patient's ability to pump blood to the body. This is what makes their blood pressure drop so low. We treat this condition by getting the infection under control and supporting the patient's blood pressure.
- Signs and symptoms of infection – in elderly people, one of the first signs of infection is altered mental status. If the patient seems 'off' or 'not themselves', it is worth notifying a healthcare provider to prevent a worse situation.
- The patient will need to ensure he is drinking plenty of fluids and practicing good hygiene to prevent urinary tract infections. He may also consider cranberry juice.
- If receiving a PO course of antibiotics – be sure to take the full course and notify HCP of any adverse reactions.

MATERNAL NEWBORN

Nursing Case Study #15
(Maternal Newborn)

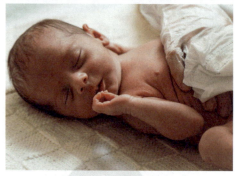

Pathophysiology:
In pregnancy GTPAL is used to identify the total number of pregnancies, including current pregnancies (Gravidity), the number of pregnancies that have gone to term (Term), the number of pregnancies that have been preterm (Preterm), the number of abortions (Abortion), and the total number living (Living). GTPAL is read as Gravidity, Term, Preterm, Abortion, and Living. For example, I'm currently 39 weeks pregnant, I have had two children born at 37 and 35 weeks. I lost 3 pregnancies prior to 12 weeks and have 2 living children; this would be read G6 T1 P1 A2 L2.

Patient:
Luisa, 25 years old, is a 37-week pregnant patient who presents to triage with abdominal and back pain. She says she thinks she is in labor because her contractions are regular and about 10 minutes apart. Her electronic health record indicates she is G3 P1 A1 and she is followed by a local obstetrics and gynecology office. She states she thinks she may be in labor but "has not seen any fluid."

*** Test your knowledge by referencing the answer key at the end of this study!*

Critical Thinking Check #1   *(Bloom's Taxonomy: Understand)*
What does G3P1A1 mean in regard to this patient?

Critical Thinking Check #2   *(Bloom's Taxonomy: Understand)*
What does the triage nurse understand labor to be in a pregnant woman?

MATERNAL NEWBORN

Nursing Case Study #15
(Page 2)

Vital signs are as follows:

- **BP** 150/94 mmHg **SpO2** 98% on room air
- **HR** 91 bpm and regular Pain 2/10 at rest, 8/10 when she reports a contraction
- **RR** 12 bpm at rest, 24 bpm when she reports what she thinks is a contraction
- **Temp** 36.8°C

Critical Thinking Check #3 *(Bloom's Taxonomy: Analyze)*
Which vital sign is most concerning to the nurse? What should they do regarding this vital sign?

The nurse decides to take the patient's blood pressure manually which gives a reading of 130/82. Therefore, the patient is admitted to the labor and delivery unit.

SBAR report is given and Luisa's admission for labor is started. She is placed in a convertible birthing bed with a fetal monitor attached to her abdomen.

Critical Thinking Check #4 *(Bloom's Taxonomy: Understand)*
What is the monitor called? What is it for?

Luisa progresses through an uneventful labor with her significant other at the bedside. She does not want any pain control and eventually delivers her newborn son, to be named after his father, Santiago.

MATERNAL NEWBORN

Nursing Case Study #15
(Page 3)

Critical Thinking Check #5 (Bloom's Taxonomy: Evaluate)
At the time of birth, how would staff evaluate Santiago?

They determine Santiago is healthy enough to be placed on his mother's chest to promote bonding and encourage breastfeeding. The staff takes him from his mother after a few minutes and she asks why.

Critical Thinking Check #6 (Bloom's Taxonomy: Evaluate)
What are staff doing when they remove Santiago at 5 minutes old?

Santiago weighs 3550 grams and is 50.6 cm long. Luisa and Santiago, Sr. ask what that is in pounds and inches so they can tell family and post on social media.

Critical Thinking Check #7 (Bloom's Taxonomy: Apply)
How does the staff respond to this?

Luisa and Santiago (referred to as a "mother-baby couplet") are moved from the labor & delivery unit to the postpartum care unit as per protocol. The staff takes the newborn to the nursery for an evaluation. Luisa wants to know what they are looking for and if her son is healthy.

Critical Thinking Check #8 (Bloom's Taxonomy: Apply)
How should the nurse respond?

MATERNAL NEWBORN

Nursing Case Study #15
(Page 4)

While the infant is being evaluated in the nursery, postpartum staff come in and assess Luisa. She wants to know why they keep feeling her abdomen and asking her about bleeding. She says, "I thought everything went OK. Why are you always checking on me?"

Critical Thinking Check #9 *(Bloom's Taxonomy: Evaluate)*
What is the best answer for Luisa?

The mother-baby couplet is set to be discharged home after a few days. It turns out that Luisa has no living children as her first pregnancy ended in stillbirth and her second was a miscarriage. She holds Santiago and is tearful as staff prepare to educate her for going home. She says, "I am so afraid I will hurt him or not do stuff right. Why do I keep crying? This is overwhelming."

Critical Thinking Check #10 *(Bloom's Taxonomy: Apply)*
Should the nurse address this? What may help the transition from a postpartum unit to home?

Answer Key:

 Critical Thinking Check #1:

- Gravida 3 (number of pregnancies), P 1 (number of live or stillbirths) A 1 (number of abortions [induced] or fetal demises before 20 weeks' gestation). So, Luisa could have 3 pregnancies and no live children (due to stillbirth) or 1 live child. She may have had an abortion or a miscarriage. Note: if A is 0 it may be omitted.

MATERNAL NEWBORN

Nursing Case Study #15
(Page 5)

Answer Key: Continued

💡 **Critical Thinking Check #2:**

- Labor is defined as regular and painful uterine contractions that cause progressive dilation and effacement of the cervix. Normal labor results in descent and eventual expulsion of the fetus.
- Interpreting labor progress depends on the stage and phase:
- First stage: The time from onset of labor (i.e., when contractions started to occur regularly every three to five minutes for more than an hour) to complete cervical dilation (noted when first identified on physical examination)
- Phases: The first stage consists of a latent phase and an active phase. The latent phase is characterized by gradual cervical change, and the active phase is characterized by more rapid cervical change.
- Second stage: The time from complete cervical dilation to fetal expulsion.
- Third stage: The time between fetal expulsion and placental expulsion.
- Lack of fluid indicates that the rupture of the membranes (amniotic sac) has not occurred yet

💡 **Critical Thinking Check #3:**

- This blood pressure may indicate pre-eclampsia ("Preeclampsia refers to the new onset of hypertension and proteinuria or the new onset of hypertension and significant end-organ dysfunction with or without proteinuria after 20 weeks of gestation or postpartum in a previously normotensive woman").
- (Hypertension denotes a rise in systolic blood pressure of 30 mmHg or more and a rise in diastolic blood pressure of 15 mmHg or more from baseline)
- The end-organ dysfunction is evaluated by looking at certain criteria: proteinuria, platelet count, serum creatinine, liver transaminases, pulmonary edema, new-onset and persistent headache unresponsive to analgesics, and visual symptoms."

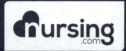

MATERNAL NEWBORN

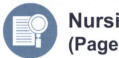

Nursing Case Study #15
(Page 6)

Answer Key: Continued

 Critical Thinking Check #4:

- "Tocodynamometry provides contraction frequency and approximate duration of labor contractions" and measures both fetal heart rate and maternal contractions. It is placed externally to watch both mother and baby as labor progresses." There are also internal devices that can be placed on the fetus within the mother to monitor fetal heart rate.

Critical Thinking Check #5:

- "Staff asks three questions. The answers are used to determine whether the newborn is admitted to the normal nursery (neonatal level of care 1) or requires a higher level of care (neonatal level of care 2, 3, or 4)
- Is the newborn's GA ≥35 weeks?
- Does the newborn have good muscle tone?
- Is the newborn breathing or crying?"

Critical Thinking Check #6:

- Checking an Apgar score ("Apgar score — The Apgar scores at one and five minutes of age provide an accepted, universally used method to assess the status of the newborn infant immediately after birth. Although data from a population-based study reported that lower Apgar scores of 7, 8, and 9 versus 10 were associated with higher neonatal mortality and morbidity, the Apgar score should not be used to predict individual neonatal outcomes as it is not an accurate prognostic tool
- The following signs are given values of 0, 1, or 2, and added to compute the Apgar score. Scores may be determined using the Apgar score calculator.
- Heart rate
- Respiratory effort
- Muscle tone

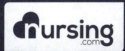

MATERNAL NEWBORN

Nursing Case Study #15
(Page 7)

Answer Key: Continued

- Reflex irritability
- Color

- Approximately 90 percent of neonates have Apgar scores of 7 to 10 and generally require no further intervention. These neonates usually have all of the following characteristics and can be admitted to the level 1 newborn nursery for routine care:
- Gestational age (GA) ≥35 weeks
- Spontaneous breathing or crying
- Good muscle tone
- Pink color
- Also, they record length, weight, head and chest circumference.

💡 Critical Thinking Check #7:

- A size chart may be available for staff to convert from metric to English measure and electronic health records may convert these values. But it is key that nursing staff know how to convert mathematically.
- 50.6 cm/2.54cm per in = 19.9 inches (long)
- 3550 gm x .0022 gm/lb = 7.8 lbs or 7 lbs 12.8 oz. Alternatively, the nurse can convert gm to kg (3550 gm = 3.55 kg) then 3.55 kg x 2.2 lb/kg = 7.8 lbs (the 10th place is multiplied by 16 oz to convert to ounces i.e., 0.8 x 16 = 12.8)

💡 Critical Thinking Check #8:

- Staff frequently (per protocol) assess a postpartum mother for possible complications. A good acronym for this assessment is BUBBLE which is essentially a focused head-to-toe (working from top to bottom) assessment.
    - B – breasts (tenderness, size, shape, etc.)
    - U – uterus (is it firm, boggy? This is done by feeling the fundus and

MATERNAL NEWBORN

Nursing Case Study #15
(Page 8)

Answer Key: Continued

- massaging if necessary. This is to help assess for a serious postpartum complication – maternal hemorrhage)
- B – bladder (is mom voiding? Is there distension or difficulty urinating? This is also a good time to discuss self-peri-care)
- B – bowel (is mom constipated? She may need a stool softener to ease discomfort)
- L – lochia (quality, quantity of postpartum bleeding).
- You could also add an "L" for legs to check for swelling, Homan's sign, etc.
- E – episiotomy (if this was done, it should be assessed for bleeding or hematoma. Use the REEDA acronym to remember what to look for {Redness, edema, ecchymosis, discharge, approximation)

Critical Thinking Check #9:

- "By pressing on your abdomen, we are assessing your fundus to ensure that the uterine muscle is properly contracting, which prevents bleeding. Similarly, we are evaluating how much you are bleeding to verify that there are no complications after delivering your baby."

Critical Thinking Check #10:

- Explain that hormonal changes (for mother) are to be expected at this time but reassure her that discharge criteria have been met. Maybe explain, "In the United States, because of concerns that early discharge could adversely affect maternal and infant health outcomes, both state and federal governments passed postpartum discharge laws in the late 1990s (Newborns' and Mothers' Health Protection Act [NMHPA]) to prevent extremely short hospital stays. In general, these laws require insurance plans to cover postpartum stays of up to 48 hours for infants born by vaginal deliveries (96 for c-sections). The impact of legislation ensuring insurance coverage for a

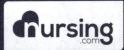

MATERNAL NEWBORN

Nursing Case Study #15
(Page 9)

Answer Key: Continued

- minimum of 48 hours has increased the LOHS of newborn infants and their mothers and appears to have decreased neonatal readmission rates and emergency department visits."
- Also, providing resources for education and follow-up will help ease anxiety. Always be prepared with whatever resources the facility and/or OB/GYN practice provides. There may be support numbers or websites available and those should be provided to the mother as appropriate.

HEART FAILURE

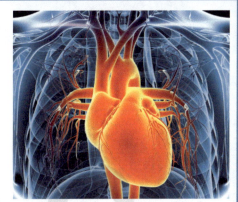

Nursing Case Study #16
(Heart Failure)

Pathophysiology:
In heart failure, the heart does not pump effectively. This can occur because of many reasons but usually, because there has been damage to the heart tissue. The heart is not able to pump enough fluid forward so fluid then backs up. This fluid backup increases work on the heart as it tries to keep up and cannot.

Patient:
Mr. Jones, a 69-year old male, presents to the Emergency Department (ED) after visiting his primary physician complaining of general fatigue for 4 days, shortness of breath, and abdominal discomfort. Mr. Jones's medical history includes hypertension and coronary artery disease. He had a previous 90% LAD blockage and 50% RCA blockage with stent placements in both.

***Test your knowledge by referencing the answer key at the end of this study!

Critical Thinking Check #1 *(Bloom's Taxonomy: Apply)*
What initial nursing assessments need to be performed for Mr. Jones?

Critical Thinking Check #2 *(Bloom's Taxonomy: Analyze)*
What diagnostic tests do you anticipate being ordered by the provider?

Upon further assessment, the patient has crackles bilaterally and tachycardia. A chest X-ray shows cardiomegaly and bilateral pulmonary edema. An ECG revealed atrial fibrillation. His vital signs were as follows:

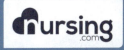

HEART FAILURE

Nursing Case Study #16
(Page 2)

- **BP** 150/72 mmHg Urine Yellow and Cloudy
- **HR** 102-123 bpm and irregular
- **BUN** 17 mg/dL
- **RR** 24-32 bpm
- **Cr** 1.2 mg/dL
- **Temp** 37.3°C
- **H/H** 11.8 g/dL / 36.2%
- **Ht** 175 cm
- **LDH** 705 U/L
- **Wt** 79 kg
- **** BNP** 843 pg/mL

Mr. Jones was admitted to the cardiac telemetry unit. Mr. Jones states that this weight is approximately 3 kg more than it was 3 days ago.

Critical Thinking Check #3 (Bloom's Taxonomy: Analyze)
What is the significance of Mr. Jones' weight gain?

Critical Thinking Check #4 (Bloom's Taxonomy: Analyze)
What medications do you anticipate the provider ordering for Mr. Jones? Why?

About three hours after admission to the telemetry unit, Mr. Jones's skin becomes cool and clammy. His respirations are labored and he is complaining of abdominal pain. Upon physical examination, Mr. Jones is diaphoretic and gasping for air, with jugular venous distension, bilateral crackles, and an expiratory wheeze. His SpO2 is 88% on room air and it was noted that his urine output had been approximately 20 mL/hr since admission. His BP is 190/100 mmHg, HR 130 bpm and irregular, RR 43 bpm.

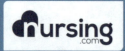

HEART FAILURE

Nursing Case Study #16
(Page 3)

Critical Thinking Check #5 (Bloom's Taxonomy: Apply)

What nursing interventions should you perform right away for Mr. Jones?

Critical Thinking Check #6 (Bloom's Taxonomy: Analyze)

Describe what is happening to Mr. Jones physiologically.

Critical Thinking Check #7 (Bloom's Taxonomy: Analyze)

What medications should be given to decrease Mr. Jones's preload? Improve his contractility? Decrease his afterload?

Mr. Jones was transferred to the CCU for hemodynamic monitoring and aggressive therapy. His Central Venous Pressure (CVP) was found to be 19 mmHg, Cardiac Output was 4.5 L/min, Cardiac Index was 2.3 L/min/m2. He has been placed in high-fowler's position, and his SpO2 is now 96% on 4L nasal cannula. Mr. Jones received Furosemide 80 mg IV and Digoxin 0.5 mg IV.

Critical Thinking Check #8 (Bloom's Taxonomy: Comprehension)

What is the expected outcome of administration of Furosemide? Digoxin?

HEART FAILURE

 Nursing Case Study #16
(Page 4)

Answer Key:

Critical Thinking Check #1:

- Full set vital signs
- Heart sounds
- Lung Sounds
- Pulses
- Edema
- Skin condition (color, temperature, etc.)

Critical Thinking Check #2:

- Chest X-ray
- 12-lead EKG
- Echocardiogram
- BNP
- Cardiac Enzymes

Critical Thinking Check #3:

- 1 kg weight gain is equal to 1 liter of weight gain. This means Mr. Jones has gained 3 liters of fluid (as volume excess) in just 3 days.
- This likely means that there is a new onset or exacerbation of heart failure

Critical Thinking Check #4:

- Diuretics – he is volume overloaded and it is affecting his lungs. Diuretics can help relieve fluid retention by promoting excretion of water from the kidneys.
- Beta-Blockers – his blood pressure is high and his heart rate is fast. The beta-blocker can help slow this down and relieve some of the workload of his heart

HEART FAILURE

Nursing Case Study #16
(Page 5)

Answer Key:

Critical Thinking Check #5:

- Place into High Fowler's position
- Apply oxygen
- Administer any PRN medications available for blood pressure (like hydralazine or metoprolol) if criteria are met
- Notify the provider

Critical Thinking Check #6:

- Because his heart cannot pump blood efficiently to the body, the blood is backing up into the lungs. This causes pulmonary edema. His pulmonary edema is so severe that he is struggling to breathe and struggling to oxygenate appropriately.
- His heart is trying to work extra hard to compensate for the low cardiac output, that's why his blood pressure and heart rate are so elevated. This is perpetuated by the RAAS.
- We also see that his kidneys are not being perfused as his urine output has decreased

Critical Thinking Check #7:

- Preload – diuretics (furosemide, bumetanide, spironolactone), ACE inhibitors (captopril, enalapril), ARB's (losartan, valsartan), ARNI's (sacubitril/valsartan)
- Contractility – Inotropes (dobutamine), cardiac glycosides (digoxin)
- Afterload – Beta Blockers (metoprolol, carvedilol), vasodilators (hydralazine, nitrates)

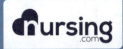

HEART FAILURE

 Nursing Case Study #16
(Page 6)

Answer Key: Continued

 Critical Thinking Check #8:

- Furosemide – should see increase in urine output and decrease in respiratory symptoms – may also see a decrease in any peripheral edema
- Digoxin – decrease heart rate and increase the force of contraction – should see evidence of improved peripheral perfusion.

R v L HEART FAILURE

Left Ventricle is unable to pump blood into the systemic circulation causing a "back-up" into the pulmonary circulation.

Right Ventricle is unable to pump blood into the pulmonary circulation causing a "back-up" into venous circulation.

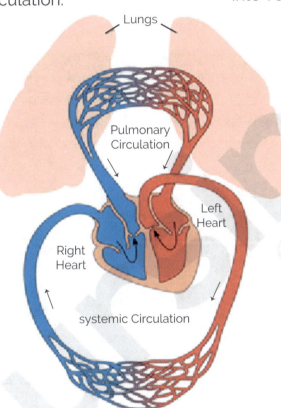

Symptoms:
- Shortness of Breath
- Dyspnea on Exertion
- Crackles
- Pink-Frothy Sputum
- Cyanosis
- Fatigue
- Orthopnea
- Tachycardia
- Confusion
- Restlessness

Symptoms:
- Jugular venous Distention
- Fatigue
- Ascites
- Anorexia
- GI distress
- Weight Gain
- Dependent Edema
- Venous Stasis

ACUTE KIDNEY INJURY PATHOCHART

PATHOPHYSIOLOGY

Acute Kidney Injury is sudden onset renal damage caused by either decreased perfusion to the kidneys (prerenal), damage to the kidneys themselves (intrarenal), or obstruction of flow out of the kidneys (postrenal). This leads to impaired ability of the kidneys to filter toxins from blood, regulate fluid & electrolytes, or maintain acid-base balance. Usually reversible, may resolve on its own, but can lead to permanent damage if not reversed quickly.

ASSESSMENT FINDINGS

- Azotemia - ↑ BUN/Creatinine
- ↓ Glomerular Filtration Rate (GFR)
- Decreased urine output in oliguric phase
- Signs of volume overload
- Metabolic acidosis
- Electrolyte abnormalities
  - ↑ Potassium
  - ↓ Sodium
  - ↑ Phosphate
  - ↓ Calcium

DIAGNOSTICS

- BUN, Creatinine Levels
- Glomerular Filtration Rate
- Clinical Findings

NURSING PRIORITIES

- Balance Fluids &
- Manage Elimination Needs

THERAPEUTIC MANAGEMENT

- Identify & treat cause
- Daily weights
- Restrict fluid intake
- Monitor urine output
- Patient may require dialysis
- During diuretic phase, replace fluids & electrolytes

MEDICATION THERAPY

- Diuretics
- Inotropes and Vasodilators to improve renal blood flow

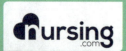

STROKE SYMPTOMS BY LOCATION

Middle Cerebral Artery
Contralateral facial weakness
Contralateral hemiplegia
Ataxia
Speech impairments (L brain)
Perceptual impairments (R brain)
Visual deficits

Anterior Cerebral Artery
Weakness of foot and leg
Sensory loss in foot and leg
Ataxia
Incontinence
General "slowness" lack of spontaneity

Basilar Artery
Impairment of consciousness
Visual loss
Pupillary abnormalities
Midbrain, thalamic, occipital, and medial lobe infarction
Bilateral sensory and motor dysfunction

Brain Stem
Blood pressure deregulation
Respiratory failure
Difficulty swallowing
Difficulty balancing
Double vision

Posterior Cerebral Artery
Midbrain Syndrome
  Third nerve palsy
  Contralateral hemiplegia
Thalamic Syndrome
  Chorea
  Hemisensory disturbances
Visual deficits
Visual hallucinations
Memory problems

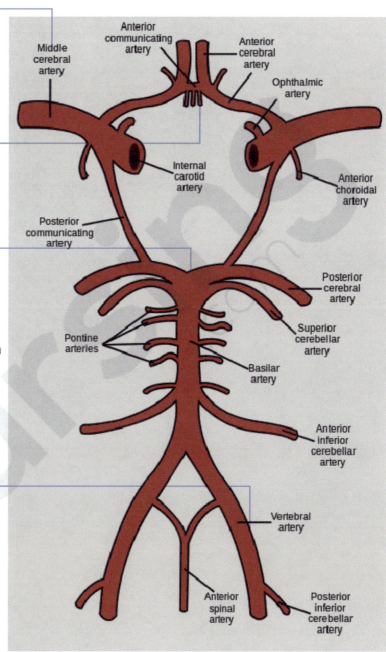

4 STEPS TO CRITICAL THINKING

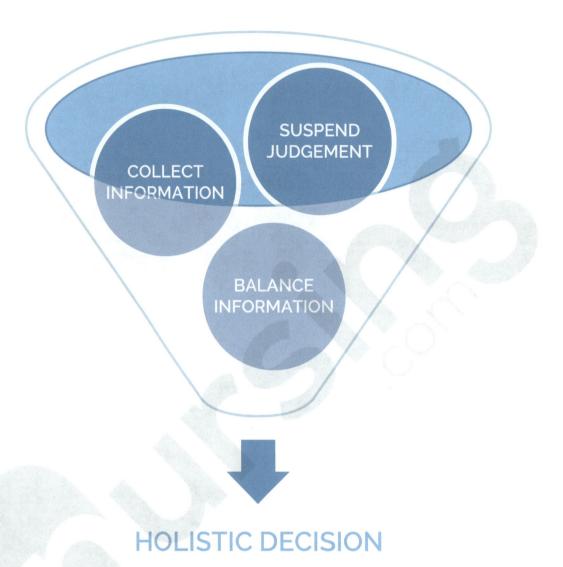

- Suspend ALL Judgement
  - Don't allow yourself to decide right away.
  - Look beyond the obvious.
  - Avoid bias.
- Collect ALL Information
  - Have you considered all options?
  - "Data Mining"
- Balance ALL Information
  - What's important?
  - Apply a value to each data point.
  - Does this achieve the desired result for my patient?
- Holistic Decision
  - Make a decision

Made in United States
Troutdale, OR
04/02/2024